CNA PRACTICE QUESTIONS

Copyright © 2018

All rights reserved.

No part of this book may be reproduced, stored in a retrieval system, or transmitted in any form or by any means, electronic, mechanical, photocopying, recording, scanning, or otherwise, without the prior written permission of the publisher.

Disclaimer

All the material contained in this book is provided for educational and informational purposes only.

No responsibility can be taken for any results or outcomes resulting from the use of this material.

TABLE OF CONTENTS

INTRODUCTION 4

CNA PRACTICE TEST 1 6

CNA PRACTICE TEST 2 62

CNA PRACTICE TEST 3 93

CNA PRACTICE TEST 4 117

CNA PRACTICE TEST 5 148

CNA PRACTICE TEST 6 189

CNA PRACTICE TEST 7 234

CNA PRACTICE TEST 8 255

CONCLUSION 289

INTRODUCTION

The CNA written Exam portion uses a multiple-choice format to test your knowledge of nursing concepts. You have 90 minutes to complete 60 questions.

This is what is covered in the written part of the exam:

There are 19 areas that will be tested on this exam. They are:

1. Safety
2. Personal care
3. Range of motion
4. Mental health
5. Vital signs and testing
6. Anatomy and physiology
7. Nutrition

8. Daily living activities
9. Body mechanics
10. Data collection
11. Aging process
12. Cultural and spiritual needs
13. Client rights
14. Infection control
15. Ethical and legal issues
16. Communication
17. Role of CNA
18. Responsibility of CAN
19. Medical terminology

CNA PRACTICE TEST 1

(60 Questions)

This is the first of our free CNA Practice Tests. In preparing our Certified Nursing Assistant Practice Testes, we ensure a strict adherence to the NNAAP standards, which is employed in several other CAN state tests also. There are 36 questions on physical care skills, 16 questions on the role of the nurse aid, and 8 questions on psychosocial care skills. We understand the importance of CNA exams – the reason behind the preparation of this test.

With this test, we hope you can prepare adequately and pass your exams at your first attempt, thus beginning your journey to your career without delay.

Question 1

One of the following responsibilities is NOT expected of a nursing assistant:

A. Bathing a resident or assisting in the process

B. Dispensing medications

C. Cleaning the room of a resident

D. Using an ice pack (if directed to)

Answer is B

The dispensation of medications is not expected of a nursing assistant. This role is left to personnel with the relevant license, like the RNs, LPNs, and others.

Question 2

Battery towards a patient may come in which of the following forms:

A. Cleaning the glasses of the resident by the nursing assistant.

B. Seeking permission, by the nursing assistant, from the resident before proceeding to touch or help them bathe.

C. Bathing the resident without their consent

D. Isolation of a particular resident, by the nursing assistant, from other residents as a form of punishment

Answer is C

When the nursing assistant bathes a resident without their permission, such is considered as a battery. Isolation (Option D) is seen as a form of involuntary seclusion.

Question 3

Having detected that a resident in the facility is suffering from abuse due to several mysterious bruises, refusal to provide answers to inquiries, and

unwillingness to undergo ADLs. How best can you approach the situation as a nursing assistant?

A.   Inform the nurse assigned to care for the patient about these bruises.

B.   Inform the immediate supervisor about the situation at hand

C.   Persist in asking the resident to pinpoint the person responsible for the abuse

D.   Search for more proof that could lead to the abuser

Answer is B

Any form of abuse or suspicions of abuse in a nursing facility must be brought to the notice of the nursing assistant's supervisor. This is because the situation at hand is beyond the scope of the practice of a nursing assistant. It is not good enough to wait or notify the nurse about the abuse; this may hinder the resident from getting the needed help in time.

Question 4

One of the following is an example of MRSA; which?

A.   A resistant strain of bacteria that withstands antibiotics treatments

B.   A resistant strain susceptible to treatment with antibiotics

C.   A mnemonic to remember how to act in the event of a fire in the facility

D.   A group of activity guidelines made to ensure the safety of residents

Answer is A

MRSA is an acronym for Methicillin-Resistant Staphylococcus Aureus, and it is not vulnerable to several antibiotic treatments.

Question 5

Infection is best averted using which of the following methods?

A. Applying standard precautions in resident care and treatments

B. Cleaning the hand with an antiseptic hand rub before applying resident care and treatments

C. Ensuring safe contacts with body fluids by using gloves

D. Washing the hands regularly

Answer is D

The most reliable and easiest method of averting infections is to wash the hands regularly. The other options are regarded as supportive measures.

Question 6

One of the following is considered an important part of care when bathing a resident?

A. Cleaning the resident's perineal area before their face

B. Ensuring better circulation by using cool water for bathing

C. Allowing residents participate in the care to give them a sense of independence

D. Handling all the care tasks for the resident so that the resident can save some energy

Answer is C

When a nursing assistant allows a resident to take part in the caring process, they are giving them a form of autonomy, while increasing their self-esteem. Using cool water instead of the comfortably warm water is unaccepted, likewise cleaning the face after the perineal area.

Question 7

Among all the possible skin care measures a nursing assistant can apply to a resident, which of the following is correct?

A. The nursing assistant does not begin perineal care except in the presence of a second staff member

B. Reporting an identified unbalanced red area on the sacrum of the resident to the nurse

C. Applying a talcum powder below the resident's abdominal folds

D. Applying a prescription ointment on the order of the nurse

Answer is B

Any red pressure spots discovered on the resident's skin must be immediately reported to the nurse by the nursing assistant, without applying any prescription ointments. There is no need for a second staff member for perineal care, and Talcum powder is not fit for this situation.

Question 8

<u>One of the following checks must be completed before shaving a resident by the nursing assistant?</u>

A.   The instructions on shaving that concern clotting issues or problems

B.   Heart condition history of the resident

C.   The presence of a personal razor of the resident

D.   Any history of refusing ADLs by the resident

Answer is A

The resident's plan of care contains important shaving instructions. The nursing assistant is expected to check and be informed about any clotting-related issues, as well as the importance of an electric razor over a traditional razor for shaving.

Question 9

One of the following is a probable symptom of fecal impaction?

A.   Dark urine

B.   Excessive Flatulence

C.   Stool leakage; usually small and watery

D.   Pains around the abdomen

Answer is C

Fecal impaction is best explained as a watery leakage of stool around a blockage, and it is also called referred to as bowel obstruction.

Question 10

Dyspnea explains a situation where a resident experiences difficulty with which of the following processes?

A. Urinating

B. Breathing

C. Swallowing

D. Defecating

Answer is B

When a patient finds it difficult to breathe, the condition is called Dyspnea.

Question 11

Which of the following statements is right about Alzheimer's residents?

A. Increased appetite as the condition becomes more severe

B. Inability to re-orientate the residents because of their ease of forgetfulness

C. Probable misperception, but not hallucinations

D. Keeping to a specific routine to keep away overstimulation and confusion

Answer is D

Alzheimer's patients are helped significantly when a specific routine is adhered to. It is not strange for them to experience a sharp drop in appetite as well as recurring hallucinations. However, a regular reorientation is necessary.

Question 12

All but one of the following aspects are wrong concerning making an occupied bed. Which is wrong?

A. Temporarily putting the dirty linen on the floor, pending when clean sheets will be fixed on the bed

B. Lower the bed to the lowest level when the procedure is complete

C. Not raising the rails of the bed, except when it is absolutely required

D. Having new sheets mitered is no longer accepted

Answer is B

To ensure safety, it is best that the bed is lowered to its lowest level. It is fine to miter the corners of the sheets; same for raising the side rails. However, you should never keep dirty linens on the floor.

Question 13

A nursing assistant must report a pulse rate as high as:

A. 45
B. 98
C. 82
D. 64

Answer is A

Once a pulse is outside the 60-100 range, a nursing assistant should inform the nurse as a matter of urgency, to ensure the safety of the resident.

Question 14

Which of the symptoms below depicts hypoglycemia?

A. Tachycardia
B. Polyuria
C. Dry and hot skin
D. Sweating

Answer is D

When a patient sweats more than usual, and experience confusion and tremors, such patient is most likely suffering from hypoglycemia.

Question 15

Which of the guidelines below is correct concerning residents who have a hearing impairment, except one?

A. Involving family members to ensure that they get the message you are trying to pass across

B. Attempting to improve understanding by speaking in a loud voice

C. Using the writing method instead of speaking

D. Maintaining a clear voice and slow speed when talking to the resident

Answer is D

When you speak clearly and slowly, residents with hearing issues stand better chances of hearing and understanding the message.

Question 16

The best interpretation of an order asking a resident to be in High Fowler Position for every meal is:

A. Making the resident lay on their stomach for twenty minutes before eating

B. Setting the bed of the patient at an angle of 30 degrees, while slumping the patient slightly over the left

C. Setting the patient's bed at a 60-degree angle with the feet propped up.

D. Setting the bed of the resident to an angle of 90 degrees, while the patient is sitting up

Answer is D

For a patient in High Fowlers, they must be sitting straight up in bed, the patient's bed must be positioned at a 90-degree angle, thus providing enough support for the patient.

Question 17

The best equipment to wear for protection while changing an incontinent patient is?

A. Gown plus gloves

B. Gown plus mask

C. N-95 mask

D. Mask, gown, and gloves.

Answer is A

A nursing assistant will be adequately protected by wearing just the gown and gloves.

Question 18

One of the symptoms listed below relates to a resident suffering from an infection. Which?

A. Tented skin

B. Pale skin

C. Abrupt start of confusion

D. Aphasia

Answer is C

For residents suffering from an infection, especially older clients, there is a high possibility of an abrupt start of confusion. Conditions like pale and tented skin are typical for older clients. However, Aphasia is common to patients suffering from a stroke.

Question 19

The nursing assistant knows that the term "NPO" means:

A. Bed rest only

B. The absence of the need to record oral temperatures

C. No oral ingestion

D. Liquid diet

Answer is C

"Nil Per Os" is the full form of the Latin abbreviation - NPO, and it means "nothing by mouth" in English. An NPO means that no oral medication, fluids, or food must be given to the patient.

Question 20

One of the following actions by a diabetic patient warrants an immediate report to the nurse:

A. Patient refusing to eat

B. Patient experiencing numbness in their feet

C. Patient combing their hair without being directed to do so

D. Patient's refusal to conclude a will

Answer is A

When a diabetic person refuses to eat, a nursing assistant must report to the nurse. Ordinarily, a diabetic patient should eat regular foods that will ensure their blood sugar level is stable or close to stability. Numbness in feet is considered as a neuropathic feeling, and it is common to diabetic patients.

Question 21

Bed rest requires turning the patient every:

A. 2 hours
B. 1 hour
C. 6 hours
D. 8 hours

Answer is A

After every two hours, a patient undergoing bed rest must be turned. This is to maintain the integrity of the patient's skin.

Question 22

A nursing assistant will use one of the pulses below in the process of acquiring vital signs:

A. Popliteal
B. Radial
C. Brachial
D. Femoral

Answer is B

The best and most easily accessible location for taking a pulse is the radial pulse.

Question 23

In a situation where a nursing assistant is assisting residents feed in the dining room, and a resident unexpectedly leaves their seat and start clutching their throats and coughing silently simultaneously, which of the following ways is the first and best way to proceed?

A.   Check if the resident is choking by asking them

B.   Call 911

C.   Commence an instant CPR

D.   Commence the Heimlich maneuver

Answer is A

An initial assessment is the most important; the nurse assistant must check if the resident is choking or not. If the patient can answer, then it means the trachea still allows the passage of air. If they answer in the affirmative by nodding, but unable to speak, the next action should be an immediate commencement of the Heimlich maneuver. Note that Heimlich isn't suitable for patients that cannot speak or cough.

Question 24

A new roommate has just been assigned a room where a client already stays. While the new roommate was in the bathroom, the client asks the nurse, "Did you bringing her here because she is sick too?" What is the best response to this question as a nursing assistant?

A. "I can't say exactly, I'll check her chart and get back to you."

B. "I think its best you ask her."

C. "You are both here for the same purpose!"

D. "It is not appropriate for me to share that information with you."

Answer is D

According to HIPPA, it is incumbent on a nursing assistant to keep the health information of a client confidential.

Question 25

You are faced with a situation where a resident with Alzheimer's suddenly wakes up one morning and starts showing signs of heightened confusion. As a nursing assistant, the best way to complement the client's normal gastrointestinal tract function is by:

A. recording the client's intake and output
B. ensuring that the client brushes their teeth
C. making the client visit the bathroom
D. helping the client to get through to their family members

Answer is C

The best way to proceed will be to make the client visit the bathroom, as this will encourage a bowel movement which will, in turn, support GI tract health. It may be difficult for a disorganized client to interpret and act on the urge on his or her own.

Question 26

A client with type two diabetes requests your assistance in cutting her toenails. As a nursing assistant, how best will you proceed?

A. Get the client a safety clipper

B. Inform the nurse of the client's request

C. Verify the blood glucose level of the client before proceeding to trim her toenails

D. Consult the chart for orders from the physician on the cutting of nails

Answer is D

Most times, there are specific instructions from the physician on trimming of nails for diabetic clients. Thus, it is best to check the chart before anything.

Question 27

How best is Insomnia prevented?

A. Making the client take one apple daily

B. Urging the client to have multiple naps per day

C. Urging the client to have numerous walks around the facility every day

D. Urging the client to stay in bed all day

Answer is C

When a client walks or engages in similar physical activities, there are higher chances of having a restful and relaxing night.

Question 28

After confessing to taking a sip of hot tea, the temperature of an elderly client was determined by a nursing assistant to be 100.6 degrees F. From the actions listed below, which one is the most appropriate for this situation?

A. Waiting for not less than 15 minutes before taking the temperature again

B. Accepting the temperature reading, and subsequently recording it in the chart

C. Scolding the client for not seeking permission before taking the hot tea

D. Taking an axillary temperature instead of the normal temperature

Answer is A

A waiting period of 15 minutes is enough to ensure an increased accuracy for the temperature of the mouth. Going for an axillary temperature will reduce the chances of having an accurate reading.

Question 29

Having discovered that a client under her is suffering from a severe "foot drop," the nursing assistant in question will most likely find which of these devices with the client?

A.   A wedge

B.   A lift (mechanical)

C.   Positioning boots

D.   Two additional pillows

Answer is C

Positioning boots are known to make the feet dorsiflexed, such that there is no contractures or discomfort.

Question 30

After taking the blood pressure of a client to be 82/43 and the client complaining of dizziness, the nursing assistant is expected to:

A. Proceed by checking the pulse of the client
B. Inform the nurse about the developments
C. Insert the readings in the chart
D. Order the client to take more fluids

Answer is B

Every case of symptomatic low blood pressure must be reported to the nurse as a matter of urgency and for an extensive investigation.

Question 31

"Abduction" as a motion term describes:

A. A movement that keeps the extremity away from the body

B.   A movement that keeps the extremity closer to the body

C.   A movement that takes the extremity above the body

D.   A movement that takes the extremity below the body

Answer is A

When you "abduct," it means you are moving the extremity closer or toward the body.

Question 32

Which of the following is the best way to deal with a client with spirituality needs?

A.   Speak to the client about why he or she chooses a certain faith

B.   Offer the client everything necessary for a warm bath every morning

C. Help the client in getting to the chapel of the facility every Sunday

D. Regard any object of religion in the room of the client like any other

Answer is C

Every client is entitled to their religious stance. A nurse assistant must be supportive, and any object of religion seen in their room must be handled and treated with respect.

Question 33

One of the following is a part of the correct body mechanics that relates lifting clients?

A. Ensuring that the spine is curved
B. Waist bending
C. Knee bending
D. Trying not to seek assistance

Answer is C

Knee bending is the only correct body mechanics in the list. All others are not safe and must not be attempted.

Question 34

Hepatitis can be indicated mainly by which of the following?

A. Hypertension
B. Hyperglycemia
C. Jaundice
D. Hypotension

Answer is C

It is very common for clients who have Hepatitis to exhibit Jaundice also referred to as the yellowing of the skin.

Question 35

Out of the aspects of care listed below, which is the most important concerning a confused client?

A. Having a periodic check of the blood sugar of the client

B. Asking for the client's name

C. Ensuring the client does not leave their room

D. Performing periodic reorientation of the client using calendars, clocks, and family mementos

Answer is D

The essential aspect of care is consistent patient reorientation. When a nursing assistant restricts the movement of a client to his or her room, this could prompt agitation, and the reaction is same when you ask for their name (which they may find difficult to recall).

Question 36

Hospice care applies to what type of client?

A. A client suffering from kidney conditions

B. A client battling cancer

C. A client that is terminally ill

D. A diabetic client

Answer is C

Hospice care is suitable for clients that are terminally ill. The hospice care works well in relieving pain instead of curing a disease.

Question 37

For Cheyne-Stokes respiration to occur in a client, such client must:

A. Have had severe respiratory problems in the past

B. Be unconscious

C. Be on a recovery journey from an asthma attack

D. Be close to death

Answer is D

Increased respiration, labored breathing, and intermittent apnea (i.e., not breathing at all) are the characteristic features of Cheyne-Stokes respiration. Thus, reporting such conditions to the nurse is essential, especially if they are exhibited by a client who is not expected to show them.

Question 38

Which of the following solutions is best suited for a day room client having a panic attack?

A. Encourage the client to take slow and deep breaths

B. Helping the client to talk about the panic attack

C. Helping the client express their feelings in words

D. Seeking to find out the cause of the panic attack from the client

Answer is A

It is best that the nursing assistant make the client feel at ease first by encouraging them to take deep and slow breaths. Counting backward from 100 can also be of great help. When a client has panic attacks, they are most likely unable to discuss anxious situations or describe those stressful and frustrating feelings. Likewise, they are unable to focus on anything apart from the symptoms. Thus, it is difficult for such client to talk about what really caused their attack.

Question 39

A resident doing any of the following is showing an orthopneic position:

A. Sitting in a chair while maintaining a straight back

B. Sitting on the side of the bed while leaning forward over a bedside table

C. Walking with the aid of a cane

D. Laying on the stomach while keeping their face to the side

Answer is B

The leading role of an orthopneic position is to aid breathing. Thus, a position that makes the client lean forward will improve the flow of air into the lungs.

Question 40

Which of the following possible breakfast items for a resident contains the highest amount of potassium?

A. Eggs
B. Cantaloupe
C. Toast
D. Strawberries

Answer is B

There is a very high potassium content in the Cantaloupe melon. The same is found in bananas and dark leafy greens.

Question 41

A nursing assistant that wants to assist a client with a weakness of the left side arising from a CVA will position the cane where?

A. The client's front

B. The client's left side

C. The client's right side

D. Out of the reach of the client

Answer is C

The best position to place the cane is on the client's strongest side so that it can provide adequate support for the weak side.

Question 42

Cardiopulmonary resuscitation (CPR) is suitable for situations where:

A. The client shows no sign of consciousness

B. The client is unable to breathe properly

C. The client cannot breathe and has no pulse

D. The client cannot breathe but has a pulse

Answer is C

CPR is only necessary for situations where the client is not breathing and has no pulse.

Question 43

On entering the room of a resident, the nursing assistant discovers a burning fire inside the trashcan. What should be the first action of the nursing assistant?

A.   Request for help
B.   Do an immediate evacuation of the patient
C.   Attempt to put out the fire
D.   Quickly reach for the fire alarm

Answer is B

According to RACE, the acronym designed for fire situations and which means Rescue, Alarm, Contain, and Extinguish, the first option is to rescue the client and ensure their safety.

Question 44

In which of the following patient diagnoses is the long-rolling technique applicable?

A. Fracturing of the left tibia

B. Injuries of the Spinal Cord (SCI)

C. Right arm cellulitis

D. Psychosis

Answer is B

In the leg rolling technique, the legs are such that they do not cross over the midline, usually in a twisting motion. And this ensures that there is no additional damage and injury to the spinal cord, in patients already suffering from SCI.

Question 45

A client that consistently declines the urge to defecate will most likely experience:

A. Constipation
B. Incontinence
C. Insomnia
D. Poor appetite

Answer is B

When the bladder eventually becomes too full and is unrelieved, the resulting condition is Incontinence.

Question 46

One of the following grief types is viewed as a healthy and normal aspect of grieving:

A. Anticipatory
B. Complicated
C. Unresolved
D. Inhibited

Answer is A

In anticipatory grief, the grief usually starts before the actual loss and is considered a typical part of grieving. In inhibited, unresolved, and complicated grieving, there is typically no problem with recovering from the loss.

Question 47

If a client is on a clear liquid diet, one of the following must not be included in his or her diet:

A. Water
B. Tea
C. Coffee
D. Orange juice containing pulp

Answer is D

The pulp that comes with the orange juice is not seen as a clear liquid. However, other liquids like water, coffee, and tea, can be added to the clear liquid diet.

Question 48

One of the prior preparations by a nursing assistant for a client with a Foley catheter and a twice-daily ambulation order is:

A. Ensuring the bag is kept below the bladder level

B. Ensuring the bag is kept above the bladder level

C. Using a pillow sleeve to keep the bag covered

D. Confirming the ambulation order from the nurse

Answer is A

For Foley catheter patients with twice-daily ambulation order, the bag must be kept below the level of the cavity. This blocks the upward gravitational movement of bacteria into the bladder.

Question 49

To keep a patient in restraints, one of the following must be in place:

A. An approval from the administrator of the hospital

B. A permission from the charge nurse

C. Physical restraints

D. An order from the physician

Answer is D

A nursing assistant cannot apply restraints without the physician giving the order. If such is done without the physician's order, it is considered illegal, and if another person other than the physician asks that the client is restrained, it is viewed as a battery.

Question 50

How best can a nursing assistant record the amount of juice consumed by a resident that consumed a bagel and one large glass of orange juice?

A. 480 cc
B. 120 cc
C. 120 ml
D. 480 ml

Answer is D

The use of the abbreviation - "cc" is no more acceptable in the medical field. The only acceptable unit is "ml," and a large glass usually has a volume of 4980 ml.

Question 51

A certain resident on the unit is suspected to be suffering from tuberculosis, hence placed on airborne precautions. The doctor needs sputum specimens to confirm the presence or absence of the disease and has ordered the nursing assistant to collect these specimens. What is the best time for the nursing assistant to carry out this order?

A. Before the resident eats
B. After the resident eats
C. In the morning, before any other thing
D. In the night, as the last thing before the patient sleeps

Answer is C

The sputum with the highest concentration, which will provide the results of the highest accuracy, is best recovered when the patient has just woken.

Question 52

Walking into the patient's room and finding him masturbating, what is the next action for a nursing assistant?

A. Condemn the act and tell the patient to be remorseful

B. Leave the room immediately to give the patient some privacy

C. Inform the nurse-in-charge about the situation

D. Talk to the patient about the reason he is engaging in such an act

Answer is B

When a patient masturbates, it is a means of expressing their sexual health. Try to leave without making noise or causing a distraction. This is to ensure that the client is neither disturbed nor deprived of his decency and privacy.

Question 53

A patient suffering from extreme agitation is allocated to a nursing assistant, and she continually yells, screams, and attempts to bite a staff. The best thing the nursing assistant can do here is to:

A.   Introduce restraints to make sure the client stays safe

B.   Engage the client in a discussion, using a calm, authoritative, and neutral tone

C.   Distract the client using the television

D.   Restrict the patient's care to when it is necessary

Answer is B

When the nursing assistant speaks to the patent in a calm, authoritative, and neutral tone, it will calm the agitation considerably. Restraints are unfit for situations like these where pacification works.

Question 54

A client suffering from terminal illness informs the nursing assistant one morning that he has started praying every night with the hope that he will be pardoned of his sins by God of receiving divine forgiveness from God. This stage of grief is called:

A. Acceptance
B. Bargaining
C. Denial
D. Anger

Answer is B

Here, the bargain is about "forgiveness" to receive "healing," and it is a normal stage in grieving.

Question 55

When moving an immobile client from their bed to a chair, the best assistive equipment to use is:

A. Mechanical lift
B. Draw sheet
C. Gait belt
D. Wrist restraints

Answer is A

The best equipment for moving immobile or NWB clients is the mechanical lift. For clients that are PWB or FWB, the best equipment is a gait belt.

Question 56

A nursing assistant is about to start a bed bath with a patient, and right before turning the patient to rub their back, she discovers the

presence of a Foley catheter. Where is the best place to keep the catheter so that it doesn't get pulled during the bath?

A. The bed
B. The bed sheet
C. The lateral aspect of the thigh of the patient
D. The medial aspect of the thigh of the patient

Answer is C

When you secure the catheter to the lateral aspect of the patient's thigh, you are assured that it will not be pulled painfully while bathing the patient.

Question 57

A resident who has just been informed about the demise of his wife begins to lament to the nursing assistant on how life will be difficult without his partner. He says, "...this is

unbelievable! I am shocked beyond normal. I don't know what I would do without my loving wife." The best response the nursing assistant should offer is:

A. "Time is all you need to cope with the loss of your wife."

B. "I feel for you, and I am sorry for your loss. I'll be with you."

C. "Well, everyone will eventually face this situation one day."

D. "Is there a child between you two?"

Answer is B

Saying this shows that the nursing assistant understands the pain of the patient and is ready to comfort him.

Question 58

While assisting a patient with a recent condition of a right-sided stroke in the bath, a nursing assistant can best support the patient's independence by:

A. Leaving the client to handle as much of the bath as he can

B. Asking the patient to seek any help he wants

C. Help him from start to finish, so that he saves some energy

D. Encourage the patient to do as much as he can to get himself cleaned

Answer is A

The best support a nursing assistant can offer is to let the patient handle as much of the bath as he can while providing the necessary helps when required.

Question 59

After receiving the complaints of a burnt leg from a patient, due to a hot soup dropping on it, and discovering blistered and red skin, the nursing assistant can identify the type of burn as:

A. Superficial burn

B. Partial thickness burn

C. Total thickness burn

D. Serious burn

Answer is B

A partial thickness burn has the appearance discussed in the question. It is a total thickness burn when the skin appears white and waxy, and a superficial burn when the skin blotch without blisters.

Question 60

A client who has not had a bowel movement throughout the last four days will find which of the following procedures highly beneficial?

A. Endoscopy
B. Colonoscopy
C. Catheterization
D. Enema

Answer is D

When the Enema procedure is applied, the patient gets to eject the fecal contents before it can become impacted.

CNA PRACTICE TEST 2

(31 Questions)

Basic Nursing Skills

Question 1

One of the following intravenous therapy tasks is not expected to be handled by a nursing assistant. Which?

A.   Running the intravenous feed into the patient before inviting the supervising nurse for assessment

B.   Preparing the solution correctly

C.   Be available to monitor the progress of the drip and report any problems

D.   Nursing assistants have no business with intravenous processes

Answer is C

It is permissible for a nursing assistant to monitor the flow of the drop, and inform the nurse-in-charge of any unusual development. However, he or she may not initiate the feed or prepare the solution.

Question 2

If a client shows signs like chills, redness, fever, and swelling. Such a case is most likely an:

A.   Infection
B.   Food Poisoning
C.   Arthritis
D.   Allergy

Answer is A

The combination of these symptoms signifies an infection. When there is swelling, alongside redness and fever, it is a local infection.

Question 3

A resident that needs protection from self-harm in a care facility setting will need which of the following?

A. Isolation
B. Restrains
C. A close observation, 24/7
D. Extra staff

Answer is B

The only instance where restraints are allowed is when the physician prescribes them, and the only applicable case is when the resident is in the position to hurt themselves. If you isolate such patient, there are increased chances of harming themselves, and the other options of a 24/7 monitoring or an extra staff are almost not feasible due to a large number of residents to be catered for in the facility.

Question 4

All of the following are not applicable to the proper hand washing process, except?

A.   The use of antibacterial soaps

B.   Ensuring longer friction time for soaps that do not lather

C.   The use of a towel in turning off the faucet

D.   The use of friction for 15 seconds

Answer is C

Germs' spread is prevented by using a towel in turning off the faucet. The other options are not applicable to a proper hand washing procedure because it takes more than 15 seconds to achieve proper friction, and the use of only antibacterial soap may not be an option. Likewise, some soaps work best when they do not lather too much.

Question 5

Axillary reading usually is lower compared to other temperature readings. Why?

A. It is outside the body

B. The period of reading or observation is shorter

C. It goes deeper into the body

D. The readings are taken at the back of the body

Answer is A

Axillary readings are recorded from the armpit, in contrast to other readings taken from inside the body, like the ear, rectum, or mouth.

Question 6

One of the following is the right step when taking a radial procedure. Which?

A. Using the pads of two fingers; press gently on the side of the neck

B. Tripling the number of beats counted in 30 seconds

C. Counting extra 90 seconds in cases of irregular pulse rate

D. Using your fingers, press gently against the radial bone

Answer is D

In taking a radial pulse, the fingers must be placed on the inside of the wrist and against the radial bone, and this lasts for 60 seconds. Hence, the other options are wrong.

Question 7

Which of these is wrong about taking a rectal temperature?

A. When necessary; cleaning the rectum of the patient after taking the reading

B. It is possible to record a rectal temperature reading that is slightly higher than a corresponding oral temperature reading

C. To ensure the accuracy of readings, it is best to use mercury thermometers

D. In an adult, the thermometer may go 1 to 1.5 inches deep

Answer is C

As a result of the dangers posed by mercury, there has been a ban on the use of mercury thermometers in medical facilities. All other options are right concerning taking rectal temperature readings. However, for infants, the depth is less than 1 inches.

Question 8

It is possible to take a pulse in all of these areas except where?

A. The inner wrist
B. Side of the neck
C. At the back of the knee
D. Behind the head

Answer is D

You may not take a pulse behind the head, but all other locations listed in the other options are allowed.

Question 9

One of the following is wrong concerning the Heimlich maneuver:

A. You may place your hands between the xiphoid and the umbilicus of the resident

B. You should make a fist with your hands to ensure the correct application of the Heimlich maneuver

C. Apply the Heimlich maneuver instantly in residents experiencing aggressive coughing

D. You may self-perform the Heimlich maneuver if alone and choking using the back of a chair

Answer is C

The object will most likely be dislodged if the resident can still cough on their own. In instances where the resident is unable to cough or speak, you should do the maneuver instantly. Other options are right, concerning the Heimlich maneuver.

Question 10

Which of the following suggestions by a nursing assistant is wrong concerning easing the use of restraints on a resident?

A.   Knowing the triggers responsible for the resident's agitation

B.   Showing the restraints to the resident to remind them that the same will be used on them if they do not desist from such behavior

C.   Knowing which activities eases the resident

D.   Distracting or redirecting the resident

Answer is B

It is grossly inappropriate to threaten residents with restraints as a form of punishment. The only right time to use restraints is when a physician prescribes it. A nursing assistant has no say in the use of restraints on a resident. Other options are good for diffusing the use of restraints, although its effectiveness depends on the peculiarity of the situation.

Question 11

Transmission-based precautions are:

A. Acts of standard-based precautions which is binding on all residents

B. Included in standard-based precautions for residents suffering from possible or confirmed communicable diseases

C. Used only in situations of an epidemic

D. Less rigorous compared to other precautions

Answer is B

The addition of transmission-based precautions to standard-based precautions will hinder the spread of any infectious disease. Other options are wrong because transmission-based precautions are not universal; they can be more severe compared to other precautions; and is applicable in other situations, other than an epidemic.

Question 12

Which of the following is false concerning condom catheters?

A. Changing them frequently is compulsory
B. Reduced effectiveness compared to external catheters
C. Recommended for avoiding urinary tract infections
D. Works better on the area in the absence of pubic hair

Answer is B

As external catheters, condom catheters offers enhanced convenience compared to internal catheters. All other options are correct.

Question 13

You can make a resident more comfortable after helping them onto a bed pan by doing one of the following:

A. Lowering the head of the bed

B. Raising the head of the bed

C. Invite the patient's trusted loved one to help with the procedure

D. Use the television as a means of distraction

Answer is B

When you raise the head of the bed as soon as you set up the resident on a bed span, you are making them more comfortable. Television as a means of distraction may adversely affect the procedure, while other options may offer discomfort instead.

Question 14

A resident releases brown fluid from the rectum; experience excessive amounts of flatus; and feels slight cramps in the abdominal region. Such a patient is probably having:

A.   a blood clot
B.   a heart attack
C.   an enema
D.   a stroke

Answer is C

All of the options may be observed after an enema procedure. In cases where the cramps become severe, inform the charge nurse. None of stroke, blood clot, or a heart attack is associated with these symptoms.

Question 15

None of the following is enough reason to seek the attention of a charge nurse concerning the ostomy bag of a residence, except:

A. The stoma leaking pus

B. 98.8 degrees of temperature

C. A rapid increase in the amount of stool in the pouch

D. Bulging of the stoma's surrounding skin

Answer is B

98.8 degrees of temperature is nothing abnormal. However, a bulge or pus around the stoma, as well as a rapid increase in the stool, both require urgent attention of the charge nurse.

Question 16

A device having two soft plastic prongs attached to a plastic tube delivering oxygen is medically referred to as:

A.   a nasal shunt

B.   a nasal antihistamine

C.   a nasal cannula

D.   an oxygen diffuser

Answer is C

All other options, apart from C, are right. A nasal cannula is used in feeding oxygen directly to the nose.

Question 17

Pressure sores under elastic stockings in a resident with a venous stasis condition is due to:

A.   wrinkles in the elastic stockings

B. inadequacy of the elastic stockings as a treatment method

C. constant scratching of the legs by the resident

D. allergic reaction of the resident to the elastic

Answer is B

It is normal for pressure sores to cause wrinkles in bed sheets or stockings of the resident. Although various symptoms come with the other options, an article pressing against the body consistently will eventually lead to the development of pressure sores.

Question 18

In turning a patient, the catheter tube can be held firmly against pulling by taping it to which part of the patient's body?

A. knee
B. the upper thigh
C. the outer thigh
D. bed frame

Answer is B

When you tape the catheter to the upper thigh of the patient, you can rest assured that there will be neither a physical trauma nor an accidental removal of the tube. Other body parts may cause pulling and removal of the tube in the process of turning the patient.

Question 19

The urinary output measurement standard is?

A. liters
B. cups
C. milliliters
D. ounces

Answer is C

The standard for measuring urinary output is milliliters (ml). Although cubic centimeters (cc) is equal in volume to milliliters (ml) and used by some facilities, it is not seen as best practice. This is because the abbreviation "cc" can be mixed up with the abbreviation "u" (i.e., units).

Question 20

The best way to proceed if you are not sure of your ability to singlehandedly turn an obese patient during their re-positioning is:

A. Avoiding turning the client singlehandedly

B. Offer the patient something sturdy to hold onto while advising them to move on their own

C. Request the assistance of the patient's family members

D. Request the assistance of another nursing assistant

Answer is D

In this case, it is best that you should ask another assistant to help you in lifting the patient. This averts the possibility of injuring the patient or yourself if you go on to turn them on your own. You do not want to injure the family members too, so do not invite them.

Question 21

Padded side rails are best used for:

A. Restraining
B. Preventing skin breakdown
C. Keeping a resident away from injury
D. Keeping a resident in the ideal temperature

Answer is C

The best use of padded side rails is to keep the resident away from injury. All other options are wrong.

Question 22

For a patient with kidney issues, one of the following 24-hour urine values is considered outrageous, and require an immediate report to the nurse:

A.   800 cc
B.   1900 cc
C.   600 cc
D.   1400 cc

Answer is C

A 24-hour urine output outside the ranges of 800 and 2000 cc is abnormal. 600 cc of urine within 224 hours is most likely a result of a complication, and the nurse should be informed.

Question 23

If a CNA wants to record 8 ounces of milk as a standard measurement of documentation in the facility, which is cubic centimeters (cc), he or she will record:

A. 8 cc
B. 360 cc
C. 240 cc
D. 120 cc

Answer is C

Every ounce is approximately 30 cc in volume; thus 8 ounces would be about 240 cc of fluid.

Question 24

One of the following food items is questionable, if found in the tray of a patient on a strict dysphagia diet?

A. Peanut butter

B. Applesauce

C. Chocolate pudding

D. Mashed potatoes and gravy

Answer is A

Difficulty in swallowing is usually associated with patients on strict dysphagia diet; they may only consume pureed foods that are considerably thin. All foods except peanut butter are too textured and may harm a patient on a strict dysphagia diet.

Question 25

You read "NPO" on the door of your patient. What can you deduce from this?

A. That the patient is permitted to take only liquids

B. Isolation precautions are binding on the patient

C. The patient may fall

D. The patient may not have any form of oral consumption

Answer is D

Foods or fluids via mouth is not allowed for "NPO" patient.

Question 26

A patient that shows such signs as sweet, fruity-smelling breath, a slight confusion, and low pulse is most likely suffering from:

A. Hypotension

B. Hyperglycemia

C. Hypertension

D. Hypoglycemia

Answer is B

Slurred speech, warm skin, confused or sluggish conduct, deep respirations, low pulse, and sweet or fruity-smelling breath are all signs of high blood sugar or hyperglycemia.

Question 27

One of these is a wrong action towards caring for a patient with diabetes:

A.   Relaxing the patient by giving them a thermal foot soak once a day

B.   Close observation and reporting (if necessary) of the patient's food intake

C.   Ensuring the feet of the patient are dry and clean

D.   Giving the patient enough snacks to eat throughout the day.

Answer is A

A diabetic patient may be suffering from diabetic neuropathy, which means that there is a reduced sensation in their extremities. Thus, for these patients, soaking their feet in hot water may lead to severe injuries, as they may not be able to detect the hotness of the water. Ideally, the feet of diabetic patients should always be clean and dry, and it is recommended to provide them with plenty of snacks to eat throughout the day to stabilize their blood sugar. It is also proper to observe their overall intake closely while reporting anything strange as quickly as possible to avoid large blood sugar swings.

Question 28

A fractured hip is known to:

A. Cost a fortune to rehabilitate
B. Be the most difficult injury to recover from

C. Be the injury on which the resident complains the most

D. Be the most likely injury arising from falls of residents

Answer is D

When residents' falls are reported, most situations eventually leads to a fractured hip. The resident's overall health, age, affects all other options, as well as the type of hip fracture the patient will sustain.

Question 29

As a CNA, it is expected of you to serve as an advocate for the resident(s) that you care for. The implication of this is that you:

A. Complain when something they dislike is done to them

B. Assist them to arrive at tough decisions related to their care

C. Help them to communicate their needs when they cannot do so

D. Be inquisitive about their care

Answer is C

You are the only member of the healthcare team that spends more time with the residents. Thus, you stand better chances of having close discussions with them. This close relationship may translate to friendship, and which requires you becoming their advocate. As an advocate, you assist in communicating their needs when they cannot do so.

Question 30

One of the following sites requires extra care during changing, because it may contain unintentionally discarded needles:

A. a resident's bath towels and washcloths
B. a resident's trash bag
C. a resident's bed linens
D. a resident's clothing

Answer is C

As many procedures requiring the use of needles and other "sharps" are done at the bedside, the bed linens may be a place where extra precaution is needed when changing as they may be a common site for unintentionally discarded needles.

Question 31

During a discussion with a dysphasic patient (someone who has issues with speaking), it is best not to:

A. use visual aids and other devices such as a whiteboard

B. encourage them to use all of their senses to convey their needs

C. finish what you believe they are trying to say for them

D. admire their efforts

Answer is C

Perhaps due to a neurological issue - Alzheimer's disease or stroke - or previous surgery to remove the cancer of the larynx (voice box), oral cavity, mouth, Dysphasia may develop in a patient. When this is the case, a CNA must always be mindful that the patient cannot clearly communicate anymore, although this does not in any way affect their intelligence. Thus, the assistant must not rush the patient or attempt to help them complete their words. Instead, the CNA should praise their efforts, be more patient, and try visual aids and devices in assisting the patient in communicating, while encouraging them to maximize their senses in expressing their needs.

CNA PRACTICE TEST 3

(25 Questions)

Question 1

One of the safety measures to put in place by a CNA when leaving a resident alone in his or her room is to:

A.   restrict the client's movement using restraints

B.   close the door tightly

C.   raise the bed to the highest position

D.   position the call light such that the patient can quickly get it

Answer is D

Ensuring the patient can reach the call light is an essential safety measure, as this is the only means through which the patient reaches his or her caregivers. The bed is best positioned on the lowest level, with bed rails up. Restraints must only be used on the directives of the physician.

Question 2

A nursing assistant that works in a skilled nursing facility is working in a:

A. Hospital
B. Rehabilitation center
C. Hospice
D. Nursing home

Answer is D

A nursing home is another word for a skilled nursing facility or long-term care facility.

Question 3

The type of healthcare facility most people, especially older people, visit after completing their treatment for a stroke at a hospital is a:

A. Sub-acute care center
B. Hospice
C. Respite center
D. Group home

Answer is A

The sub-acute care center is usually the next port of call for several older adults with stroke, after leaving the hospital. The sub-acute care centers or medical rehabilitation centers are known excellent post-stroke rehabilitation and restorative care and services to patients. CNAs also work in this facility, alongside other options in the list.

Question 4

A CNA is legally allowed to:

A. mentor other CNAs

B. teach other CNAs

C. Supervise other CNAs

D. none of the above

Answer is D

Mentorship, teaching, or supervision of other CNAs is never a business of another CNA. Instead, the nurse handles such responsibilities.

Question 5

You have been assigned to be in charge of the nursing home over the weekend because your director is unavailable. Knowing fully well that you are a CNA, what would you do?

A. Request for the necessary details

B. Put in your best in executing the assignment

C. Turn down the assignment

D. Inform the owner of the nursing home

Answer is C

You are not legally permitted to take on supervisory roles as a CNA. Thus, it is best that you reject the assignment, because if you proceed, you can face legal charges of unlicensed activities.

Question 6

The Hierarchy of Needs was created by:

A. Maslow

B. Piaget

C. Nightingale

D. Erickson

Answer is A

Maslow is credited with the creation of the Hierarchy of Needs, while Erickson created the framework of development tasks. Development of people was Piaget's project, and Nightingale is popularly addressed as the Mother of Nursing.

Question 7

Maslow's hierarchy levels include:

A.   physical needs, safety, security needs, love, and belonging needs, esteem needs, and self-actualization

B.   integumentary, respiratory, nervous, and cardiac system

C.   assessment, planning, implementation, and evaluation

D.   open-ended question, close-ended question, subjective data, objective data, and data analysis.

Answer is A

The correct Maslow's hierarchy levels are the physical needs, safety, and security needs, love and belonging needs, esteem needs, and self-actualization. Option C represents the phases of the nursing process.

Question 8

As a CNA in charge of Mrs. James, a notation on the nursing plan of Mrs. James that indicates, "Ambulate at least 10 yards qid" means that you need to assist the patient with ambulation at which times?

A. 10 a.m. and 2 p.m.
B. 10 a.m., 2 p.m., 6 p.m., and 10 p.m.
C. 10 a.m.
D. 10 a.m., 2 p.m., and 6 p.m.

Answer is B

The abbreviation - qid - means four times daily. Usually, these four times are 10 a.m., 2 p.m., 6 p.m., and 10 p.m.

Question 9

You've been asked by the RN to deliver the unit's collected lab specimens to the lab "...stat". This means that you should:

A.   Execute the task instantly without any delay

B.   Execute the task as soon as you can

C.   Execute the task after lunch or before your shift ends

D.   Ignore this task because it is not in your scope to do Stats

Answer is A

Stat is an abbreviation that indicates the instant execution of any task without any delay. CNAs are legally empowered to run such errands as taking lab specimens to the lab.

Question 10

One of the following groups consists of the five senses?

A. sight, smell, visual, taste, and auditory

B. touch, smell, taste, hearing, and sight

C. hearing, taste, smell, sight, and common sense

D. auditory, smell, taste, hearing, and common sense

Answer is B

Smell, taste, sight, touch, and hearing comprises the five senses. Seeing and visual means the same, likewise auditory and hearing. Common sense is never part of the five senses.

Question 11

In checking patients and residents, the senses applied by nursing assistants include:

A. touch, hearing, and sight
B. hearing and sight only
C. sight and common sense only
D. hearing and tasting only

Answer is A

Smell, taste, sight, touch, and hearing comprises the five senses. CNAs use only the touch, sight, and auditory senses in observing their patients and residents. Sight; to see if the patient is sleeping and determining their blood pressures. Hearing; to listen and hear out the concerns of the patients. Touch; to feel the skin of the patient, either it is warm or wet.

Question 12

The highest risk factor for falls among residents and patients is:

A. COPD
B. Old age
C. Middle years
D. Pneumonia

Answer is B

Falls are more prominent among patients with old age, followed by those in middle years. Falls are not in any way associated with COPD or pneumonia.

Question 13

One of the following sensory impairment puts the patients and residents at risks for falls:

A. Blindness
B. Confusion

C. Weakness

D. Aging

Answer is A

When a patient is blindness or suffers from low vision (both visual impairments), such patient is at a higher risk of falling because they are unable to see obstacles and hazards in their ways. Although weakness in muscles also increases the risk factor for falls, it is not a sensory impairment.

Question 14

Having heard the blaring of the fire alarms in your unit, you checked everywhere, and nobody in your unit is in immediate danger. What would you do next?

A. Move the patients out laterally

B. Move the patients out vertically

C.   Close the doors to their rooms

D.   Open the doors to their rooms

Answer is C

Patients' doors must be closed to ensure that smoke does not enter the rooms. Evacuation must be done only on instruction. According to the RACE procedure, the first action in the case of fire is R - Rescue, meaning that you need to rescue patients in immediate danger. Since patients in your unit are not in danger, A - pulling the Alarm comes next. Here, the alarm is pulled already, since you can hear it blaring. Thus, the next is C - containing the fire. And this is done by closing the doors, which will, in turn, contain the smoke and the fire.

Question 15

A CNA cleaning the genital area during perineal care is expected to:

A. cleanse the penis following a circular motion, from the base towards the tip

B. push back and replace the foreskin to cleanse the uncircumcised penis

C. cleanse the genital after rectal area

D. wash every area of the female resident with the same part of the washcloth

Answer is B

In perineal care, the genital area is cleaned such that the foreskin of the uncircumcised male patient is retracted. This is to avert the accumulation of magma under the foreskin, which if left uncleansed, can graduate to bacterial growth and infection. After cleaning the penis, the foreskin is now replaced.

Question 16

A patient that disregards the urge to defecate will eventually experience:

A.   Constipation

B.   Diarrhea

C.   Incontinence

D.   Hemorrhoids

Answer is A

When a patient continues to disregard the urge to defecate, there is an accumulation of feces and ultimately constipation.

Question 17

One of the following correctly represents a chain of infection:

A.   germ or microorganism, agent, reservoir, exit portal, transmission channels, port of entry, and susceptible host

B. active natural, active artificial, passive natural, passive artificial

C. optimism, weakness, immunity, and colonization

D. intrinsic, extrinsic, internal, and external transmission

Answer is A

A correct cycle of infection must include the germ/microorganism, the reservoir, the exit portal, the transmission channels, the port of entry, and the susceptible host. Option B describes the types of immunity, not infection cycle. Knowing about the chain of infection and how to break it is important, as it will enable you to stop the spread of infection. For instance, the chain of infection is disrupted at the transmission channels when you wash your hands.

Question 18

Asepsis is:

A. the absence of all microorganisms

B. the absence of disease-causing germs

C. a urinary infection

D. a pathogenic infection

Answer is B

Asepsis means the absence of disease-causing germs; whereas, the absence of all microorganisms, including spores, is called surgical asepsis. Pathogenic infection refers to a situation where pathogens, disease, or germ attack the body, while the urinary infection is a type of infection.

Question 19

Apart from emotional problems, there are several detrimental physical effects associated

with immobility, including adverse changes in cardiac, muscular, respiratory, skeletal, urinary, gastrointestinal, and skin structures. But a type of skeletal hazard of immobility is:

A.   contracture
B.   constipation
C.   loss of calcium
D.   catabolism

Answer is C

Although all options are problems arising from immobility, only loss of calcium, from bones, is an impairment associated with the skeletal system.

Question 20

An example of an emotional hazard of immobility is:

A.   Depression
B.   Dementia

C. Delirium

D. Diversion

Answer is A

Other emotional hazards of immobility, apart from depression, include poor decision making, and lowered self-esteem.

Question 21

A patient complains of chest pain and "a pounding heart." You examine the person's arm, and there is moisture. You also observe that the patient is sweating and has blue lips. What would you conclude as the patient's condition?

A. nervous and anxious

B. experiencing a panic attack

C. experiencing a heart attack

D. seeking emotional attention

Answer is C

Question 22

<u>A 78-year-old male patient has swelling or edema in his legs, and experience fluid restriction regarding his fluid intake. Having been assigned to take the weight of this patient daily, and with these signs, you would say he is suffering from?</u>

A. Diabetes
B. Dementia
C. Congestive heart failure
D. Contiguous heart disease

Answer is C

The symptoms exhibited by and the type of care given to this patient are indicative of congestive heart failure (CHF). Patients with the CHF condition also have dependent edema of the legs. There is an excessive volume in their blood. Thus there is a fluid intake restriction, coupled with a low salt diet. The daily weights are necessary to know the extent of water weight gain or loss per day.

Question 23

A grief is considered "healthy" or "normal" if it is an:

A. Anticipatory grief
B. Complicated grief
C. Unresolved grief
D. Inhibited grief

Answer is A

Anticipatory grief is normal; it is the grief felt before the loss or death of someone. Complicated grief, inhibited grief, and unresolved grief, are all unhealthy or abnormal types of grief.

Question 24

A family has just lost a loved one. According to one of the members, their culture frowns at leaving a dead person alone before they are buried. However, your hospital policy stipulates that all bodies must be deposited in the morgue of the hospital. As a CNA, what is the best way to handle this situation?

A. Explain the facility's policy on dead residents to the family and then implement them

B. Informing the nurse about the situation

C. Getting in touch with the primary care provider of the diseased patient to ask for advice

D. Transferring the deceased to an empty room and staying with the body yourself.

Answer is B

It is important that as a nursing assistant, you uphold the cultural needs of patients, and this should be exemplified by reporting such situation immediately to the charge nurse. The nurse may be able to go with the demands of the family concerned, based on their culture and customs.

Question 25

A small fire just broke out in a small trash can close to the lobby of the nursing home. There are no residents, staff, or visitors in immediate danger, and you have pulled the alarm. What would you do after this?

A. If possible, put out the fire safely without any harm
B. Flee from the fire
C. Use a blanket to cover the fire
D. Exit the floor after opening the windows

Answer is A

For any fire outbreak, the procedure to follow is RACE. R (Rescue) is the first step; A (Alarm) comes next; then C (Contain); and finally, E (Extinguish). In this case, there is nobody to rescue, so the R is out. You have pulled the alarm (A), and since the fire is small, it is already contained (C). The next thing expected of you is to extinguish (E) the fire. Never open the windows during a fire outbreak, and do not try to cover a trashcan fire with any material, including a blanket, as they will all likely burn.

CNA PRACTICE TEST 4

(40 Questions)

Question 1

A nurse that took a pack of bandages from the stockroom of the facility to treat her son at home has committed:

A. negligence
B. false imprisonment
C. theft
D. aiding and abetting

Answer is C

There are legal and ethical aspects to theft; however, it entails taking an item belonging to another person. Here, the nurse has taken a pack of bandages owned by the facility and not her, so it is theft. An act of negligence occurs when a nurse causes patient harm by not giving them adequate care or no care at all. When a patient is forcefully restrained from moving freely, it is called false imprisonment. A nurse that knows about an unlawful act and ignores it has committed aiding and abetting.

Question 2

A CNA that accepts his or her limitations has demonstrated which of the personal qualities below:

A. Caring
B. Dependability
C. Accountability
D. Honesty

Answer is D

By accepting his or her limitations, as well as knowing his or her job duties and being accountable for his or her actions, the CNA has demonstrated a personal quality called honesty. When a CNA shows serious concern for the safety and wellbeing of the patient, such assistant is caring. Dependability is the faith a nurse has in his or her assistant to come to work and care for patients, while accountability is performing your duties as expected of you while reporting all matters arising to your immediate supervisor.

Question 3
All of the following are verbal communication forms, except?

A. speaking clearly
B. asking questions that are open-ended
C. not making eye-contact
D. seeking clarifications to what was heard

Answer is C

Verbal communication involves speaking. All the options, except C, require talking. Avoiding eye contact, although a form of communication, is non-verbal. Non-verbal communication is usually achieved using body languages, including rolling of eyes, smiling, and crossing your arms.

Question 4

In the case where a facility seeks to transfer or discharge a patient, when is the deadline given to the resident or his or her representative before acting (either discharge or transfer).

A. 7 days
B. 14 days
C. 30 days
D. 60 days

Answer is C

A resident to be discharged or their representatives must be informed within 30 days of the proposed transfer or discharge. The rule, which is enforced by the "Residents Bill of Rights," came up after the American Hospital Association issued "A Patient's Bill of Rights" in 1973. According to the act, a facility is allowed to discharge or transfer a patient on medical grounds; for their well-being and that of other patients; or for inability to fund treatments. However, this does not apply to Medicaid patients.

Question 5

An elderly patient who has Parkinson's disease may show one of the following signs:

A. Inability to stand
B. Inability to stoop
C. Inability to walk
D. Inability to learn new skills.

Answer is D

Severe conditions associated with Parkinson's disease include arthritis or muscle tremors, which may impair walking, standing, or stooping abilities. When patients find it difficult to stand or walk, they are more likely to fall and sustain serious injuries that will get them hospitalized.

Some of the abilities of an older adult, which will not be affected by Parkinson's disease, include learning ability, and the aging process.

Question 6

Persons of age 85 and above are likely to die from which of the following primary courses?

A. fall-related injuries

B. cancer

C. hypertension

D. strokes

Answer is A

Individuals aged 85 and above has injuries from falling as their primary cause of death, and it is the second primary cause for individuals aged 65 and above. When people grow older, they experience deteriorations like poor eyesight, which is the reason elders find it challenging to walk around in the dark. Mobility is another factor that is negatively affected by aging; elders usually have less stability with their feet.

Question 7

The most appropriate description of MRSA is:

A.   a viral condition occurring on the skin, and which infects the nerve path of the patient

B.   a skin rash developing due to an attack by tiny mites

C.   a bacterial infection which results in skin seeping and blistering

D. skin disease, usually life-threatening, and which uses the blood stream as a medium for dispersion

Answer is D

MRSA is a skin disease - a life-threatening disease dispersed via the bloodstream. It is easily communicable, and may spread very rapidly throughout the entire population of a nursing facility may be affected. The skin rash that occurs as an aftermath of tiny mites' infestation is called scabies, while the nerve path of the patient is usually the main target in the viral skin condition called Shingles.

Question 8

When bathing a patient, there are two major goals associated with skin care. They include:
A. enhancing sleep and preserve the skin

B.   reduce the amount of oil on the body, and getting rid of body sweat

C.   getting rid of pathogens and ensuring comfort

D.   skin inspection and enhancing blood circulation

Answer is C

When bathing a patient, the two primary goals are to get rid of pathogens present on the skin and promote the patient's comfort. With the increase in age comes a reduction in the amount of oil produced by the skin; thus, the purpose of bathing is not to get rid of oil. Maintenance of patient's appearance, getting rid of body sweat, and enhancing blood circulation are not achievable via bathing. However, an assistant gets to inspect the skin of the resident during the bathing process.

Question 9

The best way to provide a comatose patient with oral care every few hours is by:

A.　helping in cleaning the dentures of the patient, while swabbing their mouth and mucous membranes

B.　keeping the patient's head turned to the side while using the right equipment in swabbing their mouth and mucous membranes

C.　opening the patient's mouth gently and brushing their teeth

D.　seeking the permission of the patient before proceeding with the oral care with the right equipment

Answer is B

Being comatose infers that the patient is unconscious, which makes it impossible for them to give permission or participate in their oral care.

However, you must always ensure that the head of the patient is turned to the side, as this prevents them from aspirating while using the right equipment to swab their mouth and mucous membranes. When comatose patients breathe, it is mostly through their mouths. Hence, periodic oral cares are required to keep their mouth well-hydrated.

Question 10

Which of the following is not a physical sign of pain that a patient can exhibit?

A Tachycardia

B Hypotension

C Tachypnea

D Dyspnea

Answer is B

Every option in the list is a physical sign, except hypotension or low blood pressure. Hypertension, i.e., high blood pressure is a physical sign; Tachycardia, a condition of increase in pulse, is also a physical sign, alongside dyspnea (difficulty in breathing), and tachypnea (increased respiration). Other possible physical symptoms of pain include moaning, grunting, crying, or sweating.

Question 11

To take the radial pulse of a patient, the part of the body that is of interest to you will be:

A. Neck
B. Behind the ear
C. Apex
D. Wrist

Answer is D

Radial pulse is present only on the wrist. Apex is the site for an apical pulse. For residents with heart conditions, the radial pulse should last for about a minute, and during this time, you should listen to the resident's heartbeat before recording the pulse rate.

Question 12

One of the following is not allowed when recording your observations about a patient:

A. signing your name

B. scratching out errors

C. making amendments

D. writing with red ink

Answer is D

Red ink is not allowed for recording patients' observation. The permissible ink colors are black and red. You are required to sign your name and title to all the data recorded. Mistakes are normal, but they should not be scratched out, nor erased with a liquid eraser.

Question 13

The correct way to place a patient in Sim's position is to place them:

A.   on their side while positioning the two arms in front of the patient

B.   on their side while positioning their undermost arm at their back

C.   on their back while placing the arms at their sides

D.   sitting up while leaning over their overbed table.

Answer is B

A patient in Sim's position must be positioned on their side, while their undermost arm is placed at their back. Option A is the lateral position, while C describes the supine position. Orthopneic position involves sitting a patient up while leaning over their over-bed table.

Question 14

The part of the body used in taking the tympanic membrane temperature of a patient is:

A. the ear
B. the axilla
C. the anus
D. the mouth

Answer is A

The patient's ear is the body part involved in taking a tympanic membrane temperature. Axilla is for axillary temperature; the anus for rectal temperature; and the mouth for oral temperature.

Question 15

While checking the radial pulse of a patient for the first time, you recorded 45 BPM as their pulse reading. What would you do next?

A.   Recount the pulse for another 60 seconds

B.   Inform the nurse of the patient

C.   Go ahead to record the observed pulse rate on the chart

D.   Take the blood pressure of the patient

Answer is A

An irregular pulse rate of 50 BPM or less requires you to recount the pulse for another 60 seconds. If the reading is still the same after the second count, you should inform the nurse in charge instantly, to avert any danger. The right position to place a patient before taking their radial pulse rate is the supine position.

Question 16

One of the following best describes what is expected when measuring the blood pressure of a patient for the first time:

A. to measure the blood pressure of the two arms, while recording the reading of the second arm as the baseline

B. to measure the dominant arm and record the measurement on the facility form

C. to ask the patient for their most-preferred arm and use the same for the initial measurement

D. to measure the blood pressure of the two arms while recording the reading of the first arm as the baseline

Answer is A

Question 17

The process of applying Condom catheter involves:

A. Leaving very little space between the penis and the catheter

B. Leaving a space of one inch between the penis and the catheter

C. Circling the penis using tape, to ensure the catheter is secured

D. Taping the catheter to the lower abdomen of the resident

Answer is B

A one-inch space is required between the catheter and the penis during the application of a condom catheter. Encircling the penis, using a tape, may lead to the tourniquet effect. Hence, it must be avoided. But you can secure the catheter by applying the tape in a spiral direction instead. Securing the catheter is done by taping the catheter to the inner thigh, and not the abdomen of the patient.

Question 18

In feeding a blind patient, you can try all the following except?

A.   Telling the patient about the food they will be eating

B.   Pacing the bites given to the patient, to save energy

C.   Giving the patients liquid to sip

D.   Avoid talking so that you don't disturb the patient's meal

Answer is D

You are not expected to keep mute when feeding a blind patient, because your failure to interact with them socially while eating takes away their satisfaction. Let them know what they will be eating, and space the bites to conserve energy. You should also give them liquids to sip.

Question 19

One of the following is a prerequisite for communicating with patients suffering from auditory impairment:

A. Placing yourself to the patient's side
B. Speaking in a high tone and slowly
C. Speaking only clear and short statements
D. Increasing the background noise

Answer is C

Short and clear statements are important when talking to auditory impairment patients. You should also try to stay directly in front of the patient while speaking, and ensuring that your voice is calm and in a low tone while decreasing the background noise. Only talk about things such that they do not get confused.

Question 20

A dysphasic patient has challenges with:

A. Breathing
B. Thinking
C. Walking
D. Speaking

Answer is D

A dysphasic patient cannot speak correctly, and this may be due to Parkinson's disease, cancer, Alzheimer's disease or stroke. The patient, although finds it difficult to talk coherently, can correctly understand you. Being dysphasic doesn't affect intelligence. You must show patience, compassion, and respect when dealing with them.

Question 21

One of the following is not a non-verbal communication:

A. Laughing at a funny joke by the patient

B. Eyes-rolling in response to the inabilities of a patient

C. Congratulating a patient

D. Hugging a patient

Answer is C

Non-verbal communications are executed using body languages like eyes rolling, smiling, and hugging. Verbal communication, on the other hand, involves speaking. Thus, congratulating someone requires speaking some words, making it a verbal communication.

Question 22

A nursing assistant who seeks to be a team player may accept:

A. Harassment

B. Battery

C. Hazardous duties

D. Constructive criticism

Answer is D

Being a team player involves accepting constructive criticism in good faith. Such criticism may come in the form of a superior's feedback, and if taken the right way, the performance and job satisfaction of such a nursing assistant can be significantly improved. In instances where a nursing assistant feels he or she is facing situations that threaten their safety or wellbeing, the supervisor should be notified immediately.

Question 23

A waste matter is considered hazardous when they are:

A. contaminated with blood
B. contaminated with chemical agents
C. potent enough to cause infections
D. identified as hazardous materials

Answer is C

Any waste matter that can cause infection is considered hazardous. Such wastes may contain blood alongside other body fluids. Any contaminated materials must be kept away in a marked biohazard container, for safety.

Question 24

A patient that is crying is experiencing what level of pain?

A. 0
B. 2
C. 4
D. 5

Answer is D

Tears signal a level 5 pain. Level 0 means the patient is not in pain, while level 5 indicates the pain is high enough to bring tears.

Question 25

One of the following needs does not increase with age:

A. the need to sleep
B. the need to void
C. the need to eat
D. the need to defecate

Answer is A

The need to have a good sleep increases with age, rather than decreasing. Thus, an elderly patient will require the same quality of sleep any other will, and as such, they must be allowed to rest well and take consistent naps. Unlike sleep, the need to eat depreciates with age, likewise the need to defecate.

Question 26

One of the following approaches, if taken with your patient, is right:

A. Criticism
B. Discouragement
C. Prevention
D. Apathy

Answer is C

The preventive approach is right between nursing assistants and patients, and this may entail preventing them from harm or becoming immobile or weaker. Criticism, discouragement, or indifference are unacceptable as possible approaches by a nursing assistant, as they do not improve the health of the patient.

Question 27

One of the following statements is RIGHT concerning a female patient perineal care:

A.   Starting the genital area washing from the perineum

B.   Washing the genital area using a washcloth without any soap

C.   Back to front movement while cleaning the genital area

D.   Using a fresh washcloth in rinsing the genital area

Answer is D

Always use a fresh and clean washcloth in rinsing the genital area. You should also use a soapy washcloth and not a soap-free washcloth. The genital area should be washed from front to back, and not back to front. The urinary meatus is the starting point, not the perineum.

Question 28

The best position for a patient undergoing oral care is the:

A. Supine position
B. Sim's position
C. Orthopneic position
D. Fowler's position

Answer is D

The Fowler's position entails raising the head of the patient's bed, which in turn positions them in an upright position. This position is suitable for oral care because it ensures that the patient is not choked during the process. Any other position apart from this puts the patient at the risk of choking and makes the process difficult for you.

Question 29

All of the following are parts of denture care, except:

A. Using tepid or cool water in rinsing or cleaning the dentures

B. Carrying the dentures to the sink for cleaning using your gloved hand

C. Using a paper towel to line the sink, thus reducing the risk of breaking the dentures

D. Storing the dentures in a denture cup containing clean water

Answer is B

It is wrong to carry the dentures of the patient to the sink for cleaning using your gloved hand. Instead, you should place them in a denture cup first before transporting them to the sink. Cool or tepid water must always be used to rinse, clean, and store dentures.

Question 30

The care for dementia entails all of the following except:

A.   Ensuring the room of the patient is uncluttered

B.   Avoiding arguments or disputes with the patient

C.   Calming and reassuring patients that are suspicious

D.   Varying the routines of the patients

Answer is D

Memory loss, confusion and inability to perform tasks are the main issues faced by patients who have dementia. Thus, varying the patient's routines is out of the line, as it will only add to their confusion. Leaving the room of the patient uncluttered or avoiding disputes or arguments with the resident are not included in proper dementia treatments.

CNA PRACTICE TEST 5

(40 Questions)

Question 1

As a nursing assistant who has just witnessed a patient spilling water on the hall floor, and another client walking down the same hall, what would you do?

A. Ignore the spill

B. Inform the nurse

C. Clean the spill

D. Call housekeeping

Answer is C

Leaving the spill can lead to falls, which is known to lead to severe complications and injuries, particularly among patients that are very old or weak. There is the need for every member of staff to stay alert for potential hazards such as spills while attending to the situation immediately. However, if the spill contains body fluid or blood, it is essential that you follow the protocol for decontamination and also wear a Personal Protective Equipment (PPE).

Question 2

When moving a patient, most of the patient's weight should be supported by which body part of the nursing assistant?

A. Shoulders
B. Wrists
C. Legs
D. Back

Answer is C

The position of the nursing assistant should be such that he or she supports the clients most weight using his or her legs. When in this position, the nursing assistant must keep their back straight, without turning or twisting. If they have to bend, they should do so at the hips and not the waist.

Question 3

While shaving your client, the electric shaver you are using suddenly starts sparking and smoking. What would you do first?

A. Finish the shaving with the shaver of a roommate

B. Inform the nurse in charge immediately

C. Quickly finish the shaving

D. Unplug the shaver

Answer is D

As a nursing assistant, you should always put the safety of the patient first. You should unplug any malfunctioning device to stop the sparking and smoking. Leaving such a device may lead to a fire outbreak if an oxygen source is close by. You should never use personal items of a client for another.

Question 4

A comatose oral care requires which equipment?

A. toothpaste
B. toothbrush
C. toothette/mouth swab
D. all equipment above

Answer is C

A client in comatose is unconscious; they cannot assist or participate in their oral care. Thus, the nursing assistant needs to take extra precautions that will prevent aspiration or choking during the care. With the patient's head turned to the side and the bed head lowered, clean the teeth and gums gently with a separate moist toothette or mouth swab for every part of the mouth. When done, wipe the mouth of the client, then raise the bed head to the original position.

Question 5

You are walking with a patient limited to movement on a wheelchair, and you suddenly hear the facility's fire alarm system go off. This resulted in the client becoming unnecessarily excited. What would you do in such a situation?

A. Lock the wheelchair of the patient before proceeding to check the environment for smoke

B. Calm the client and take them to somewhere safe

C. Start searching for help while leaving the client on their own

D. Discarding the wheelchair and carrying the client to somewhere outside the facility

Answer is B

According to the RACE procedure, the first action in the case of fire is R - Rescue, meaning that you need to rescue patients in immediate danger; A - pulling the Alarm comes next. Here, the alarm is pulled already, since you can hear it blaring. The next is C - containing the fire. And this is done by closing the doors, which will, in turn, hold the smoke and the fire. Then there is E - extinguishing the fire. This can be done using a handheld extinguisher if the fire is small to ensure your safety and the feasibility of an escape route.

Question 6

According to the nursing care plan, you are to transfer a patient using a mechanical lift, but

you noticed a sudden agitation by the client. What would you do?

A. Go-ahead to place the client in the lift

B. Unlocking the wheels so that the lift can move with the client

C. Lift the client but without using the mechanical lift

D. Ask for assistance in moving the client

Answer is D

Even though a patient doesn't cooperate as expected, their safety still comes first. In this situation, it is best that you request a co-worker to assist you to ensure that the patient stays safe. If after this, there is no improvement in the agitation of the client, inform the nurse in charge before doing anything else.

Question 7

One of the following is essential when taking an oral temperature:

A. Placing the thermometer under the tongue

B. Lubricating the thermometer with a suitable lubricant

C. Placing the thermometer under the arm

D. Placing the thermometer in the rectum

Answer is A

An accurate oral temperature reading is only possible when the client has not taken anything hot or cold for 15 minutes. Place the thermometer under the client's tongue; if it is a digital thermometer, there will be a beep, signaling the registration of the client's temperature. If it is a glass thermometer, you will see the line no longer moves after registering the reading. In adult patients, any temperature above 38 degrees C is considered a fever, while it is 37.5 C in children.

Question 8

How would you convert six ounces of juice to milliliters (ml)?

A.   6 x 15 ml
B.   6 x 5 ml
C.   6 x 10 ml
D.   4 x 30 ml

Answer is D

30 ml is equal to 1 ounce. While the ounce weighs slightly more, pharmacists and doctors consider the amounts equal.

Question 9

What is the first thing to do as a nursing assistant, after seeing the client's radio cord draped across a chair to reach the closest outlet?

A. Unplug the radio and tell the client not to put it on again

B. Make efforts to plug in the radio safely and correctly

C. Talk to the client about the radio as a safety hazard and keep it away from them

D. Take the client and the radio to the activities room, and allow the client to listen to the radio there.

Answer is B

Electrical safety standards of government and that of accrediting agencies must always be followed. Thus, radios, televisions, and other clients' devices must be approved based on the policies of the facility. A cord cannot cause any severe hazard, but extension cords are not allowed. As a nursing aide, you may assist the client in locating a suitable outlet to plug the radio cord, so that they may continue listening to their favorite station.

Question 10

The most important use of padded side rails is:

A. to keep the client safe from injury

B. to maintain the client's warmth

C. for restraining

D. to provide a place for connecting the call signal

Answer is A

The most important use of side rails is to keep the client from falling out of the bed, which may lead to severe injuries. If the client is confused, agitated, has a head injury, or has a history of seizures, padding the side rails can save them from further injuries or entrapment. You can make a side rail pad by using a mattress pad, and ensure that the bed is in the lowest position always.

Question 11

A device that replaces a missing body part is a:

A.   Pronation
B.   Prosthesis
C.   External rotation
D.   Abduction

Answer is B

Prostheses are devices that serve as replacements of a missing body part, either due to surgery, accidents, or birth defects. Prosthetics restore the lost function to the client and can replace missing parts of the eyes, breasts, teeth, arms, legs, and joints.

Question 12

Urinary output is measured correctly in:
A. 1 quart
B. 40 oz
C. 2 cups
D. 300 cc

Answer is D

As a metric measurement, 300 cc is the same as 300 cubic centimeters. The metric system is the adopted system of measurement for length, volume, weight, and temperature readings across the medical field worldwide. It is known for the highest level of precision it provides, which is based on units of ten.

Question 13

A catheter will not pull in the process of turning a male patient if the catheter tube is taped to:

A. the client's upper thigh
B. the client's hip
C. the client's bed frame
D. the client's bed sheet

Answer is A

The function of an internal urinary catheter is to remove the contents of the bladder into an external bag. For males, the catheter is usually a long tube with a balloon that is inflated on insertion. The draining tube must neither be bent nor pulled. The inner thigh is the only point of attachment in male patients, and the attachment is done using tape or other fastening devices. It is essential that the bag used in draining stays lower than the bladder of the client, to prevent the urine from flowing back.

Question 14

As a nursing assistant, you encounter clean, unused bed linen while checking your client's room, what would you do?

A. Take it to the nurse-in-charge
B. Keep the linen in the dirty linen container
C. Have it returned to the linen closet
D. Apply it to another client's bed in the next room

Answer is C

A linen present in the resident's room is unclean, as each room may contain pathogens and sources of possible infection, especially the objects present in such a room. It is also important to discard all supplies opened with sterile packaging.

Question 15

The role of the hormone - Insulin is:

A. To regulate the strength of the skeletal muscles

B. To regulate the heart's rhythm

C. To regulate the salt content of the blood

D. To regulate the blood sugar level

Answer is D

Insulin is essential in diabetic conditions, which arises due to the inability of the pancreas to make enough insulin that will reduce the amount of blood sugar in the system. Diabetic patients are required to have their blood levels checked daily. They must undergo treatments to remain healthy, and their treatments sometimes include insulin injections.

Question 16

You want to assist your client to walk from the bed to the chair, what would you place on the client's feet?

A. Nothing
B. Slippers with soles made from cloth
C. Slippers or shoes with rubber soles
D. Stockings or socks only

Answer is C

Slippers or shoes with rubber soles will prevent the client from fallings associated with ambulation; thus, it is fit for walking both short and long distances. Do not employ stocks, stockings, or fabric-soled slippers, as they can make the client slip and fall. Likewise, walking without any footwear can cause injuries to the foot, and this can lead to further complications in diabetic clients.

Question 17

One of these is vital during the operation of a manual bed:

A.   Ensuring the client's head is elevated at all times

B.   Folding cranks under the bed

C.   Ensuring that the wheels are locked when the cranks are folded under the bed

D.   Keeping the bed in the neutral position

Answer is B

A manual bed must always be locked. This is done by pressing down the levers on the wheels situated at the foot and head of the bed. Three cranks can be found at the end of the bed, and they are responsible for controlling the height of the bed, and lowering the feet and the head. To raise each of the section, the cranks are turned from left to right (clockwise), and counter-clockwise for lowering the parts. Once the client has been positioned, the cranks must be folded to ensure that others do not fall or trip.

Question 18

One of the following is not a fire prevention measures expected of a nurse aide:

A. Taking part in fire drills

B. Preventing clients and visitors from accessing cigarettes and matches

C. Reporting any damaged sockets or wiring in the clients' rooms

D. Knowing where fire extinguishers are situated in the facility

Answer is B

Smoking of any form is inappropriate in the facility, but this does not give a nurse aide the right to seize matches or cigarettes from anyone. The best a nurse aide can do is to get familiar with the facility's policies on smoking and smoking areas and report smoking or smokers at the designated areas. It is a responsibility of every staff to know where extinguishers are placed, as well as the actions to be taken in the event of a fire outbreak. Fire can also be averted by reporting any damaged wiring or socket promptly to the nurse-in-charge.

Question 19

The abbreviation NPO means:

A. Nothing by Mouth
B. Nothing Per Ostomy
C. Only Ice Chips Per Mouth
D. Nothing by mouth other than water

Answer is A

The meaning of the medical term - NPO - is that a client is not allowed to drink or eat anything, even water, and ice chips. It is usually prescribed for situations like before some lab work or surgery. A client with a gastrointestinal condition may be put on NPO till the doctor can discover what the cause is.

Question 20

What would you do as a nurse aide if a client that is to be moved appears too heavy, and you are not sure if you can move him or her on your own?

A. Try your luck by moving the client on your own

B. Seek the assistance of a colleague

C. Invite the family to move the patient

D. Leave the client to handle another task

Answer is B

More than one person should move objects or clients that seems too heavy. Anything contrary to this may lead to falls and injuries for both the aide and the patients.

Question 21

A nurse aide assigned to a client with a protective device (restraint) should:

A. Ensure the tightness of the protective device at all times

B. Always check the body alignment of the client

C. Remove the restraints from the client once, during his or her shift

D. Check on the client once every hour

Answer is B

A physician usually orders restraints, and when one is requested, a nursing aide must follow the necessary protocols applicable, to ensure that the client is safe. By knowing the policies on protective devices, a nursing aide can care for the client better, with regards to how and when to monitor the client, how to report the status of the client, and how to document all observations.

Question 22

A client who is still recovering from a stroke and can barely walk will need the nursing aide to help them by:

A. Standing behind them
B. Providing them with a wheelchair
C. Staying on their strong side
D. Staying on the client's weak side

Answer is D

The nurse aide must stay on the weak side of the client while walking next to them slightly behind.

He or she should be ready to support the client's weak side at any moment. For clients on a cane or walker, the nurse aide must leave space for the device. The client should avoid wearing shoes or slippers with rubber soles, to avoid traction.

Question 23

A client with a respiratory problem is best placed in which position?

A. Lateral
B. Supine
C. Prone
D. Fowler's

Answer is D

Fowler's position is the best source of relief for residents with breathing problems. This involves placing the client upright at 90 degrees while allowing the chest to expand as much as possible.

Question 24

If you are to place a signaling device close to a client that is paralyzed on the right side, how would you go about it as a nurse aide?

A.   place the device on the right side of the bed, close to the client's hand

B.   place the device under the pillow

C.   place the device at the foot of the bed

D.   place it on the left side of the bed, close to the client's hand

Answer is D

One-sided weakness or paralysis is common to stroke patients, and they find it impossible to use that side of the body, or even be aware of the side. The situation is referred to as the "one-side neglect." As a nurse aide, you must encourage the client to use the unaffected side, and the best way to do this is placing the signaling device where they can reach it when they need help.

Question 25

When a client is subjected to the Heimlich maneuver (abdominal thrusts), he or she is suffering from:

A. a blocked airway

B. impaired eyesight

C. a bloody nose

D. injuries from falling out of bed

Answer is A

For clients that have their upper airway blocked by food or an object, the first aid method for them is the Heimlich maneuver. In a situation where a client is choking or appears to be, a nursing aide must try clearing the airway quickly, after which they call for help.

Question 26

As a nurse aide, you just saw fire in one of the clients' rooms, how would you react?

A. Get the client out

B. Attempt to put out the fire

C. Inform the nurse-in-charge

D. Find a way to open the windows and doors

Answer is A

According to RACE, the acronym designed for fire situations and which means Rescue, Alarm, Contain, and Extinguish, the first option is to rescue the client and ensure their safety.

Question 27

Which is the safest way of helping a client out of bed to sit in a wheelchair?

A.   By releasing the wheel brakes
B.   By lowering the bed
C.   By lowering the two footrest pedals
D.   By placing a pillow on the seat of the wheelchair

Answer is B

A safe transfer begins with lowering the bed to the lowest, thus allowing the client to reach the floor easily when standing and pivoting to sit in the wheelchair. While doing this, the wheelchair's brakes should not be open, and the footrests completely kept out of the way.

Question 28

A nurse aide seeking to lift an object with the aid of proper body mechanics will do one of the following:

A. Holding the object away from the body
B. Bending the knees while the back is straight
C. Lifting the object with abdominal muscles
D. Keeping the two feet together and close

Answer is B

The risk of injury to the low back increases when using the back muscles, bending at the waist, twisting, or trying to lift when the load is too heavy.

Question 29

You will place your fingertips on which part of the client's body when taking their radial pulse?

A. Neck
B. Wrist
C. Elbow
D. Chest

Answer is B

Radial pulses are found on the wrist, and it is detected by placing the index and middle fingers on that empty area right below the thumb. Then some light pressure will be applied to feel the pulse. The pulses must be counted for 30 seconds and the reading multiplied by 2 to determine the pulse rate. If the heartbeat rate is irregular, increase the timeframe to 60 seconds and then record the new pulse rate in the chart.

Question 30

A good nursing aide will perform one of the following to ensure the safety of a client they are leaving alone in their room:

A.   Leaving the bed elevated, in the highest position

B.   Putting the client in restraints

C.   Closing the door tightly

D.   Ensuring that the signaling device is within reach of the client

Answer is D

The call signal of the client must always be close to them when the nursing aid is absent. Safety of the client can only be achieved by lowering the bed to the lowest position possible while keeping the bed rails up. Except you have the physician's order, you must not put a client under restraint.

Question 31

The most frequent use of physical restraints is:

A. When a roommate of the client requests for its use

B. To ensure the safety of the client and keep them from injuries

C. When a family requests for its use

D. When the resident is short

Answer is B

As devices or equipment meant to prevent the normal movement, physical restraints are only used when the physician orders it. When used without the physician's order, it is illegal, and it may harm the client or others close to them. They must not be applied to punish, inconvenience, or as a method of control.

Question 32

All of the following is a means of restraining a client, except by using:

A. a hand mitt

B. a lap buddy/tray

C. pain management

D. a sedative

Answer is C

In addition to physical restraints, there are chemical restraints too, and they work by keeping the client and others safe from harm. A pain medication is not in the restraint category.

Question 33

Water can put out a fire of which type?

A. Chemical

B. Electrical

C. Paper

D. Grease

Answer is B

Based on the materials they are extinguishing, there are various classifications of fire extinguishers. The three classes are Class A, Class B, and Class C. Class A is used for combating paper, wood, textiles, and some plastics. Class B extinguishers are used for oil, gasoline, and other flammable liquids. Class C is for electrical fires. Labels are usually affixed to each fire extinguisher, which identifies their class and subsequently what kind of fire they can combat.

Question 34

The most accurate weight of a client can be taken when?

A.   After the client has just eaten

B.   After waking up in the morning

C.   A different nurse aide takes the reading

D.   At the same time of the day

Answer is D

Weight measurement should be such that the readings are taken at the same time every day, and if possible in the morning (it is the best time). The same scale should be used for the best results, and weighing should be done after the client's first void and before breakfast.

Question 35

As a nursing aide, you discover that a client suddenly starts choking and turning blue while having their dinner. What would you do?

A.   Make the client take some water

B.   Dislodge the food by continuously slapping the client on the back

C. Remove the food tray of the client immediately, before informing the nurse in charge

D. Seek assistance in performing the Heimlich maneuver (abdominal thrusts)

Answer is D

The most appropriate response to choking is Heimlich maneuver. So in this case, seek for assistance while attempting the Heimlich maneuver. This will alert others of the emergency. For the back slap option to work, abdominal thrusts must be initiated once the food fails to dislodge.

Question 36

A quad-cane base has how many tips?

A. 4
B. 2
C. 3
D. 1

Answer is A

There are four tips on a quad-cane, and these are used in creating a broad base that supports the client during walking. The cane is placed, about an arm's length away, on the strong or unaffected side of the client with all the four tips on the ground at once. Then the client should place the weak leg forward while depending on the cane for stability.

Question 37

As a nurse aide that just discovers an unresponsive resident, what would be your next action?

A. Seek assistance from others
B. Begin compressions on the client
C. Shut the door of the room
D. Inform the family of the resident

Answer is A

The best and first thing to do in any case of emergency, including when encountering an unconscious client, is to seek help. While you attempt compressions, others can assist you with it, while some people clear the area, and some call the ambulance. People can also document the events as they happen.

Question 38

Pressure on bony prominences is best reduced by:

A. Repositioning the client every shift
B. Using a sheepskin
C. Floating the mattress of the client
D. Providing the client with several

Answer is C

Repositioning should be done at least every two hours, as this prevents the skin from breaking down. Pillows can be used in supporting the client and relieve places where skin can rub, for instance at the tailbone or between the legs. The skin should be kept dry and clean at all times. When there is a sheepskin on the wheelchair or bed, it offers the patient more padding, but not the same effect as repositioning. Any reddened part of the skin must be reported to the nurse. However, pressure sores are best reduced by floatation mattresses and special beds.

Question 39

A broken side rail is observed by a nurse assistant while making an empty bed. What would be the next action of such an assistant?

A. Inform the client of the damage and warn them to be careful on the bed

B. Tell the nurse about the broken side rail

C. Only report the side rail at the next safety check

D. Keep the side rail tied in the raised position pending when it will be fixed

Answer is B

Broken equipment must never be used for a client, and a temporary fix is for damaged equipment is not acceptable as well. The best solution is to tag the bed and ensure that no other client uses the bed, and the faulty bed be replaced immediately.

Question 40

A person who treats persons with difficulties in talking, perhaps due to stroke or other physical defects is called a?

A. Occupational therapist
B. Physical therapist
C. Registered nurse
D. Speech therapist

Answer is D

A Speech Therapist helps a client that finds it difficult to speak clearly or form words, due to strokes and related physical defects, as well as swallowing disorders.

CNA PRACTICE TEST 6

(45 Questions)

Question 1

One of the situations below is the best time for using a soft toothette:

A. In the case of a resident with dentures

B. In the case of a resident complaining of a toothache

C. In the case of a resident with a seizure

D. In the case of giving an unconscious resident mouth care

Answer is D

It is very likely for an unconscious to aspirate toothpaste or fluid. But when soft toothette is used, such risks are eliminated as they are mostly untreated.

Question 2

You have just received a call from a patient, who is just recovering from a stroke and with a left-side weakness, asking for a sweater. Where do you think the assistance is most needed?

A. His left side
B. His right side
C. At his back
D. At his front

Answer is A

Because his weak side is the left side, supporting him from the left will help him to achieve and maintain his balance. The other options are not the most suitable for supporting a client with a left-side weakness.

Question 3

As a nurse aide, you should not do one of the following when giving a patient nail care:

A. Being extra careful when trimming the nails of diabetic patients

B. Preventing dryness by applying excess lotion between fingers and toes, and on the hands and feet

C. Making the process easier and faster by soaking the hands or feet of the resident in warm water before trimming

D. Drying the fingers or toes thoroughly to ensure there is no skin breakdown

Answer is D

Lotion should not be applied between fingers and toes, as this may encourage the growth of bacteria. There are guidelines on nail trimming for each facility, endeavor to go through them and find the ones applicable to diabetic patients.

Question 4

You have just been ordered to bathe an Alzheimer's patient that had visitors in the room for the most part of the shift. How would you proceed?

A. Inform the nurse-in-charge to talk to the visitors present

B. Request the visitors to excuse the patient so that you can bathe them

C. Postpone the task till the next day

D. Ask the patient when you should return for the bath

Answer is B

Taking charge of the privacy of your patient is part of the most important duties of a nursing assistant. Likewise, you must ensure that ADLs are completed within a considerable period. With the presence of visitors for "most of the shift," it means there is no opportunity for ADLs to be executed. Thus, it is best that you request them (the visitors) to wait in another area, while you bath the patient. Relying on the decision of the patient is inappropriate in this case, as Alzheimer's patients are not fit enough to make such decisions.

Question 5

You are faced with a situation where a patient on a DASH diet takes less food and shows little interest in eating. What do you think is the next action?

A.   provide the patient with their prescribed dietary supplements

B.   talk to the patient about the problem and try to encourage them to eat

C.   arrange with the patient's family on the possibility of bringing down the patient's favorite foods

D.   inform the staff nutritionist

Answer is A

The best way to proceed would be to provide the patient with their prescribed dietary supplements. While you may make some progress by engaging the patient on the problem, it may not be enough to make them eat. On the arrangement with the family, they may not bring the foods that comply with the DASH diet. The nutritionist may be involved later, but not as the first step. By dietary supplements, we mean beverages, and these do not usually include the medications of the patients.

Question 6

A patient feeds slowly during breakfast and ends up coming late to physical therapy. What is the best way of approaching this as a nursing assistant?

A.   Postpone their breakfasts until they are done with physical therapy

B.   bring the patient to breakfast earlier than usual

C.   start feeding the patient during breakfasts

D.   taking the patient's breakfast away from them once it is time for their physical therapy

Answer is B

When you bring the patient to breakfast earlier than usual, you are expected to leave them to eat on their own. Since they came earlier than usual, it will give them more time to eat and still come for the therapy on time.

Question 7

One of the following is wrong when shaving a resident:

A.   starting from the chin and shaving upwards towards the sideburns

B.   tying a towel around the neck of the resident when giving a face shave

C.   confirming if a patient has a bleeding problem from the nurse before proceeding to shave them

D.   shaving upward on the neck

Answer is A

Option A is an incorrect technique for shaving a resident. Instead, you shave downward from the sideburns. All other options are right when shaving a resident

Question 8

One of the following challenges is not associated with residents during mealtime or eating:

A.   absence of reminders for mealtimes

B.   inability to use eating utensils properly

C. inability to chew or swallow properly

D. reduced preciseness of thirst or hunger

Answer is A

Any reputable care facility is expected to alert residents when it is mealtime, as well as feeding them via caregivers or intravenous delivery of nourishment. Except this, other options represent the usual challenges faced by residents concerning eating.

Question 9

When it comes to bathing residents, one of the following is an essential factor, but it is usually neglected by caregivers and care facilities:

A. bathing residents with water of a safe temperature

B.   using adequate body mechanics to keep the residents safe during the bath

C.   there are various bathing cultures among different cultures

D.   the need to rinse and dry the patient adequately

Answer is C

Other than when it relates to setting the care schedule of a resident, cultural differences are usually neglected when it comes to bathing residents. Other options are standard operating procedures associated with bathing residents

Question 10

One of the following may depend on the rules of the facility on residents' nail care sessions when handled by nursing aides:

A. The best sitting position of the resident during nail care is sitting in a chair, and not in the bed

B. Guidelines on cutting toenails

C. Informing the nurse of blue or pale nail beds

D. Soaking the hands or feet in water for 10 minutes before trimming

Answer is B

In some facilities, cutting toenails of residents is a task that only nurses and physicians handle. Other actions are what a nursing assistant usually do when giving nail care.

Question 11

When caring for the dentures of a resident, one of the following statements is not right:

A. Dentures are fragile, and replacements cost a fortune

B. Storing dentures in cool water is necessary

C. Residents handle their denture care, so the facility is not held responsible when things go wrong

D. Dentures can be very slippery when wet

Answer is C

It is practically impossible for most residents to do their denture care on their own properly. Other statements are quite important and correct with respect to proper care of dentures.

Question 12

When a resident cannot move around by themselves, it is important to:

A. Check them routinely for pressure sores

B. Leave them clean and dry from incontinence

C. Turn them at an interval of two hours

D. Turn them at the start of a new nursing assistant shift

Answer is D

A timeframe of a new nursing assistant shift is inadequate to save residents from having circulation-inclined problems. Other actions are important when caring for patients that cannot move on their own.

Question 13

The basic application of a Hoyer Lift is in the movement of a resident on to:

A. a stretcher
B. the chair
C. a vehicle
D. the bathtub

Answer is B

As a safety device, Hoyer Lift is best for moving patients that are unable to move on their own from their bed to a chair and back. The other applications are not the basic role of a Hoyer Lift

Question 14

AM Care or Morning Care must be given to the resident before breakfast because:

A. It reduces the growth of harmful bacteria

B. It improves the sense of well-being of residents

C. It offers a pleasant appearance and experience

D. All of the above

Answer is D

Reducing the growth of harmful bacteria, improving the sense of wellbeing of residents, and offering a more pleasant appearance are all roles of the morning care.

Question 15

In addition to safety and privacy, one of the following factors is the third important consideration when bathing a resident:

A. Quiet surroundings

B. Adequate security

C. Completing the procedure quickly

D. Reduced lightning

Answer is B

A resident that is bathing will be undressed, and consequently in a vulnerable state. Hence, in addition to privacy and safety, security is quite important. Anxiety is commonly associated with bathing and showering; thus, it must not be rushed so as not to cause injuries. The preference of the resident will determine the environment - whether silent or with music playing in the background, likewise the extent of light needed for the bath.

Question 16

A resident with a skin breakdown, tooth decay, ad a bad breath is most likely suffering from:

A. Dehydration

B. Insufficient amount of toothpaste during tooth care

C. Dry mucous membrane in the mouth

D. Excessively moist mouth

Answer is C

Yes, all these might occur due to dehydration, but the basic reason the resident is dehydrated is the dryness of the mucous membrane present in the mouth. It is also possible for a resident to have dry mucous membranes in their mouth and still stay well hydrated. An excessive moist mouth cannot give such symptoms. Insufficient amount of toothpaste may also lead to bad breath, coming from tooth decay. But the best option here is the presence of a dry mucous membrane in the mouth.

Question 17

One of the following factors, although important, is often neglected when giving residents proper hair care:

A. Age
B. Race and culture
C. Length of stay
D. The conditions of the environment

Answer is B

When it comes to residents' hair care, it is common for nursing aides to overlook race and culture. Thus, it is essential to listen and be aware of how the practices of other cultures or race may differ from your opinions on hair care. Other alternatives may influence the appearance and hair of residents, but not as much as the race and culture.

Question 18

A resident with small, watery leakage of stool is most likely suffering from which of the following:

A. a reaction to medication

B. a GI infection

C. pelvic muscle weakness

D. A fecal impaction

Answer is D

Fecal impaction is best identified when there is a watery leakage of stool around a blockage. This situation is also referred to as bowel obstruction.

Question 19

An older male adult experiencing pains will most likely exhibit one of the following behaviors?

A. insomnia

B. excessive talking

C. refusal to partake in social activities

D. refusal to drink or eat

Answer is B

When an older male adult experiences an increased pain tolerance or inability to experience pain, it usually does not affect their rest or activities. Although they may deny the pain, they exhibit signs and behaviors that portrays discomfort, and such signs include reduced appetite, refusal to partake in social activities, and insomnia. Tachycardia, a condition of an increased pulse, is a physical sign, alongside dyspnea (difficulty in breathing), hypertension (high blood pressure) and tachypnea (increased respiration).

Question 20

A resident's rest and comfort can be greatly improved by:

A. creating a quiet environment

B. pacing their ADLs, recreational activities, and visiting times to allow them to rest adequately

C. keep away all positioning devices, such that they do not disturb their sleep

D. engage them in diversion activities like music, mediation, and reading

Answer is C

Positioning devices should be used to promote comfort and rest when needed. The pacing of activities is important so that the resident does not become overtired and anxious, which can prevent relaxation. The provision of quiet, calming activities and a calm environment are also important in inducing rest.

Massaging the patient and providing emotional support during the times of discomfort can be helpful, especially when combined with the routine maintenance of the physical environment to ensure safety and security, which will in turn promote good rest and sleep.

Question 21

You've received an order from the nurse to ambulate a patient BID? What does this mean?

A. ambulating the patient once
B. ambulating the patient four times
C. ambulating the patient twice
D. ambulating the patient thrice

Answer is C

"Bis In Die" is the full meaning of the abbreviation - BID, and it means twice-a-day. Once in a day is represented by QD, while thrice in a day is represented by TID. QID means four times a day.

Question 22

Most times, the best means of showing a resident that you are listening to them is to:

A. Ask questions that keeps the conversation engaging

B. Engage them in discussions while working

C. Turn in their direction while answering their questions

D. Bring in your personal experiences on the topic of discussion

Answer is C

The best way to show that you are following the conversation is to stop, face the resident, and maintain eye contact. If you show the other options, you may dissuade the resident from continuing with the conversation.

Question 23

The most important first step when starting a procedure on a patient is:

A. to ensure that there is privacy in the immediate area

B. to record what you did in the patient's medical record

C. record the date in the patient's medical record

D. verify the identification of the patient

Answer is D

Verification of the patient's identity is the most important initial step, although other steps are correct too.

Question 24

How best would you communicate with a deaf patient?

A. by using a pen and paper or a computer system

B. by projecting your voice over background noises

C. by using a phone system that amplifies

D. by using an alarm that rings louder

Answer is A

A deaf patient requires a natural and alternative means of communication. Other options may suit patients that with slight auditory problems.

Question 25

Documenting a medical record does not involve which of the following:

A. Author identification

B. Ensuring correct spellings of words

C. Writing in pencil so that you can easily correct errors

D. Ensuring all entries are dated

Answer is C

Just like a legal document, it is important not to erase medical entries. Other options are considered as part of the process.

Question 26

Which of these notations represent an order to ensure that the affected patient avoid oral consumption of any form? NB: The patient is due for surgery the following day.

A. NKA

B. NOC

C. MN

D. NPO

Answer is D

NPO means Nothing By Mouth, and it is originally in Latin - "Nil Per Os." MN means midnight, NKA means No Known Allergies, while NOC means for the night.

Question 27

Having called his family members, a resident informed you of his decision to leave the facility without the necessary medical approval as a result of frustration. What would you do first?

A. Inform the physician

B. Contact the relatives and asking them to wait

C. Inform the facility administrator of the development

D. Inform the nurse

Answer is D

The best option is to inform the nurse FIRST before other members of the healthcare team, including the physician.

Question 28

One of the following events should be reported to the charge nurse as "STAT"?

A.   a cloudy urine

B.   a respiratory rate of 18

C.   a radial pulse of 135 and above

D.   loose stools

Answer is C

Any radial pulse beyond the range of 60 and 100 is considered as abnormal in adults. A pulse rate of 135 is beyond the normal range and should be reported immediately. 18 as a respiratory rate value is still normal, and although cloudy urine or loose stools may be abnormal, they are not to be classified as "STAT."

Question 29

You should do all of the following when entering a resident's room for the first time, except?

A. entering only after knocking and waiting a few seconds

B. presenting your licensing card to the resident

C. introducing yourself to the resident

D. addressing the resident by his or her name

Answer is B

All other options portray respect for privacy, courtesy, and personal engagement, except option A. There is no need for presenting the resident with your licensing card.

Question 30

When is it best to document the input and output of a patient in their record?

A. Every two hours

B. Early morning, noon, and late evening

C. When your shift ends

D. Only the nurse is allowed to document a patient's output and input

Answer is C

The recording must be done such that the information reflects what happened during your shift, accordingly. The totals of the inputs and outputs are expected to be recorded in the patient's record before the close of work for the day.

Question 31

A nursing assistant caring for a resident with memory difficulties is expected to:

A. Make jokes and laugh to lighten the mood of the resident

B. Leave the resident alone to reduce their agitation

C. Sit and listen to the resident while making eye contacts at intervals

D. Remind the resident of any information they find difficult to retrieve

Answer is C

Reminding such patients of their forgetfulness will only get them more agitated, and they may take your jokes and laughs as a form of disrespect. You may need to spend more time with such patients while listening and showing car; this is the best way to care for them.

Question 32

One of the following does not portray visual impairment?

A. Withdrawal of the resident from social activities they once liked

B. Residents experiencing difficulty in walking on the stairs

C. Spilling or knocking food over

D. Squinting or tilting of the head to a side to focus on a certain object

Answer is A

It is possible for a resident not to partake in a social activity that requires visual acuity, although this is not an indication of visual impairment only; other unrelated factors may be associated. The other options represent other pointers to the presence of visual impairment.

Question 33

A patient that requires a magnifying glass to read; is unable to smell smoke; uses more sugar or salt on foods; and prefers maximum TV volume when watching, is most likely suffering from:

A. Sensory impairment
B. Sensory deprivation
C. Sensory overload
D. Sensory stimulation

Answer is A

A patient that has either lost or have their use of sight, hearing, smell or taste senses drastically reduced is undergoing sensory impairment. When there is sensory stimulation or sensory overload, it means there is an enhancement of the senses, while sensory deprivation refers to an intentional removal or reduction of stimuli to the senses.

Question 34

For a resident just getting admitted into a care facility, one of the following is the most crucial step:

A. Provision of all the necessary admitting information by the family, to avoid misrepresentation of the resident

B. The family should take over the admitting process and sideline the resident, to reduce the stress involved in the difficult process

C. If the resident has strong religious beliefs, it is required that a member of his or her spiritual community be around to ensure the religious requirements are satisfied

D. The resident's information should be provided by him or herself

Answer is D

It is important that the resident participates in the admitting process by providing all the information about his or her wishes or needs. However, such information can be improved on by additions from the family, especially if the resident is not sure about the details. Also, the facility should endeavor to build a relationship with the resident so that they feel like they are part of the whole process.

Question 35

The best approach to a situation where a resident is angry and frustrated is to:

A.   Talk to the resident about how normal it is to get angered with certain things

B.   Make the resident recall the reasons or causes of their anger or frustration

C.   Try to discuss with the resident about why their reaction is apparently overblown

D. Endeavor to offer support by listening to the resident, while assuring him or her of your readiness to convey his or her concerns to the members of the healthcare team

Answer is D

To relax an angry and frustrated resident, it is best to punctiliously listen and allow him/her to vent out their frustrations, so he/she sees that you care enough to help. Other options will only aggravate the situation.

Question 36

An indwelling catheter is taped down for the following primary reasons except:

A. Stabilizing and securing the device so that there is no accidental removal

B. Reduction of the inflammation of urinary tissues

C. As a way of telling visitors or family members that the catheter is not to be removed

D. As a means of offering psychological security to the patient

Answer is C

Although the taping may seem like a way of telling family and visitors that the indwelling catheter should not be removed, such intention is not regarded as a primary reason.

Question 37

You have just been informed by your nurse of your omission of a crucial information in the charting of a resident's input for that day. The chart must have contained all of the information below except:

A. lactated ringers administered intravenously

B. a protein bar snack

C. toast with breakfast

D. tea for the afternoon

Answer is A

Only a nurse is allowed to chart intravenous fluids. Other information should be recorded in the resident's intake chart.

Question 38

A nursing assistant and a resident may not communicate effectively due to:

A. The inability of a caregiver to explain in detail the processes involved when carrying out a procedure on a resident

B. The nursing assistant ignoring the opinions or contributions of the resident

C. The inability of the resident to comprehend the information a nursing aide is trying to pass

D. All of these

Answer is D

All of the options can adversely affect communication between a resident and a caregiver individually. Their combination can even make matters worse. When you listen to a resident and take an interest in their behavior, you would be able to understand them more - even things they do not say out literally. You should also be patient and detailed while explaining procedures, and be ready to answer all their questions if they have any.

Question 39

Which of the non-verbal communication methods listed below can send the wrong message to a resident?

A. Talking slowly while facing the resident

B. Answering questions correctly, but through a slightly rude voice

C. Rendering explanations in an overtly loud voice

D. Standing with hands on the hips and lips squeezed

Answer is D

All of these indicates a positive message, except option D, which sends a negative message without saying a word.

Question 40

How would a resident likely react on receiving the news that you (a nursing assistant) criticizes a co-worker in the facility?

A. They'd feel less confident in you

B. They'd think you do not care about them

C. They would be worried

D. They'd feel validated in their feelings

Answer is C

Criticizing your fellow worker as a nursing assistant gets the resident worried because they are afraid that you might do the same to them in their absence. This type of situation is an indication o your empathy for others, and this reduces the confidence a residence has in you to be open to you or start seeing your care towards them as fake.

Question 41

When caring for a patient that is speech impaired, which of the following should you avoid?

A. Attempting to finish up their sentence when they have challenges doing so

B. Helping them with an assistive device, like a pen or paper, as this will help them communicate by writing down what they find challenging to say

C. Advise them to try gestures and other non-verbal communications instead of talking or attempting to talk

D. Stay calm, patient, and understanding while the residents attempt to communicate their needs to you

Answer is A

All of the above options will frustrate your efforts to help the resident, except option A.

Question 42

Adequate verbal communication with your resident must not involve:

A. Speaking clearly

B. Using medical jargon when communicating

C. Asking them open-ended questions

D. Trying to clarify their speech or message

Answer is B

You should avoid using medical jargon when speaking to a patient. Speak clearly, using words and phrases that your resident can understand, and ask open-ended questions that discourage yes or no answers but encourage further exploration of the resident's thoughts and feelings instead. Always make sure to clarify the message you receive by repeating what you're told back to the resident. These steps ensure good verbal communication.

Question 43

Which part of your conversation with a resident will you report to ensure their safety and well-being?

A. His or her specific requests
B. His or her likes and dislikes
C. His or her favorite activities

D. His or her favorite foods

Answer is A

Developing a good interpersonal relationship with your resident will facilitate effective communication. While you should get to know him or her as well as you can, specific conversations should be reported to ensure the well-being and safety of your resident. Reporting specific requests, evaluations, concerns about care, or safety considerations, as well as a change in condition, are examples of such conversations.

Question 44

A CNA must have all of the following excellent communication skill except:

A. Delegating
B. Responding
C. Listening

D. Documenting

Answer is A

Although there is the need to learn how to delegate as a CNA, it is not classified as an important communication skill.

Question 45

A resident tells you that he feels like he's "got a lump in his chest." An example of clarifying the message he's communicated to you would be to ask him:

A. "Let me see if I understand what you mean. You feel like you have fullness in your chest?"

B. "Tell me more about that?"

C. "Are you having any palpitations or radiation of your symptoms?"

D. "Do you feel pain?"

Answer is A

Part of effective communication is to clarify the message that has been communicated to you by your resident. This involves repeating back to him or her the information that you believe was delivered to ensure that everyone is on the same page. These questions usually start with, "Let me see if I understand what you mean…?" or "Is this what I hear you say…?".

CNA PRACTICE TEST 7

(20 Questions)

Question 1

What would you do first if one of the residents under your watch and care suddenly starts showing signs of frustration and anger, with constant complaints in loud voices?

A. Ignore the patient to show them you do not condone such behavior

B. Encourage the resident to be civil in their reactions so as not to make other residents angry

C. Speaking to the resident about their situation, and supporting them in a calming and comforting manner

D. Inform the supervising nurse of the situation

Answer is C

The best way to show that you are concerned about the needs of such resident is to offer them care and support, although they may be rude. Other options will have adverse effects on the situation or do nothing tangible to solve the problem.

Question 2

Which of the five senses leaves last in a dying patient?

A. hearing
B. taste
C. touch
D. sight

Answer is A

Although they may not communicate clearly, most patients may still hear what others are saying or what is said to them. Hearing is usually the last sense to leave a dying patient, with other senses gone in the early stages.

Question 3

How would you help a resident who has just been informed about the death of his or her love go through the grieving process?

A. By encouraging the resident to replace the sad thoughts with pleasant ones

B. By staying close to the resident and spend quality time with them; and showing willingness to listen if they are ready to talk about it

C. By sharing your experience with death with the client as well as how you survived those hard times

D. By telling the client about the inevitable nature of death.

Answer is B

Being a calm and good listener gives the resident more convenience and encouragement for them to go further in sharing their feelings with you. Other options do not help or improve the situation.

Question 4

In describing the different stages of grief an individual who has just lost a loved one goes through, Elizabeth Kubler-Ross identified which of the following as the first of the stages?

A. Denial
B. Depression
C. Acceptance
D. Anger

Answer is A

According to Kubler-Ross, the first reaction when an individual sees the reality of death is denial. After denial comes the other stages above.

Question 5

If you are to deal with a resident that is anxious or showing signs of unsettlement about their environment or a certain situation, what would be your best move?

A.   Giving them some privacy so that they can re-focus and re-group

B.   Talking to them in a calm voice and a comforting tone

C.   Attempting to distract the resident from drifting into thoughts by putting on the tv or the radio

D.   Allow more light to enter and brightening the surrounding by opening the shades

Answer is B

When you speak to them in a calm and comforting voice, you are trying to reduce the stimuli that come with such anxious times. Other options work by increasing the stimuli in the environment thus making the resident more anxious and unsettled.

Question 6

When a resident consistently shows signs of confusion during dusk, early evening, or during the night, such a resident is showing symptoms of:

A. Dementia
B. Sundowner's syndrome
C. Psychosis
D. Alzheimer's disease

Answer is B

Sundowner's syndrome involves disorientation that happens mostly at night. Although the other options involve disorientation too, they are not associated with a particular time of the day.

Question 7

How would you respond to a startling sexual comment from a resident?

A. By moving on swiftly to a new subject

B. By ignoring such comments

C. By replying with a funny comment

D. By informing the resident about your reservations towards such comments

Answer is D

In such situations, you should make it clear to the resident that those types of comments are unacceptable. With this, you are setting the clear boundary between formal discussions and irrelevancies in the future. You should also inform the supervising nurse.

Question 8

The death of a resident got his roommate worried, and he is so desperate to have a discussion about it with you. How would you handle such a situation?

A.   By sharing your experience in dealing with the loss of a loved one with the client

B.   By engaging the roommate in discussions that make him express his feelings to you

C.   By switching the topics to something more exciting

D.   By making the patient understand the inevitable nature of death

Answer is B

When you offer the resident the chance to discuss the death of his roommate and how it makes him feel, you are helping him and encouraging him to seek help when they require your counseling again.

Question 9

What would you do first, as a nursing assistant, if a resident starts to pace around his room while shouting on the top of his voice and swearing?

A. Inform the family of such resident about the situation while asking them to help

B. Telling the resident to seat and stay calm

C. Request the attention of the supervising nurse

D. Proceed to put such a resident in restraints

Answer is C

The best you can do here is to request the attention of the supervising nurse, who may have to give the patient some medications that will calm them down.

Question 10

A patient undergoing the aging process will normally experience which of these:

A. a reduction in the rate of movement of food from the digestive system
B. stiffer joints with less flexibility
C. thinner bones with reduced rigidity
D. a dip in their ability to make decisions

Answer is D

A significant drop in the ability of an individual to make decisions is more associated with diseases than to the aging process, which is a normal biological change.

Question 11

One of the following is not a cause of constipation:

A. ignoring the urge to void

B. more intestinal motility

C. diet with low fiber contents

D. refusal to take adequate amounts of water

Answer is B

The reduction in the rate of intestinal motility is known to lead to constipation, but option B, which talks about an increase in the intestinal motility rate, is the opposite. Thus, constipation cannot be the correct answer.

Question 12

All of the following indicate depression, except:

A. A dip in appetite

B. Increased interest in participating in social activities

C. Withdrawal

D. Sleeping more

Answer is B

Depression is associated with a reduction of interest in participating in social activities; it does not increase it. Thus, option B is the correct answer.

Question 13

The following are the possible ways of helping a resident deal with their impending death, as a nursing assistant, except?

A. giving the resident more alone time so that they do not feel any pressure to socialize

B.   spending more time with such resident than usual, so that you offer them the support they require

C.   being a good listener whenever they need one

D.   keeping the resident's privacy as they deem fit

Answer is A

Such residents are interested in someone that will be a great listener whenever they need one to share their feelings and fears with. By leaving them alone for most of the time, you are enforcing the feelings of isolation in the resident. Other options all offer support to the resident while respecting their wishes.

Question 14

How best can you help a resident who has just been informed of the death of his or her spouse?

A.   Be a listener and supporter whenever the client needs one

B.   Attempt to lighten up the mood of the resident by cracking jokes

C.   Inviting other residents to keep the company of the resident

D.   Attempt to change the conversation to a topic that has little or no tension

Answer is A

For someone who has just lost their loved one, there may be the need to discuss their feelings or memories as regards the great loss. You may not have to do more than just sitting and holding hands, this little gesture is enough to give them the comfort they need.

Question 15

Stress comes with the caregiving job. The following are possible ways of dealing with this stress, except?

A. Joining a new club

B. Engaging in physical activities and going outside for fresh air

C. Learning something new

D. Discussing your patients with your coworkers just to air your frustrations

Answer is D

All other options are appropriate for dealing with work stress, except option D. It is not right to discuss your patients and their challenges with your colleagues, irrespective of how therapeutic such may be.

Question 16

How would you approach a situation where a family member is angry about the unhappiness of their loved one currently at your facility?

A.   Leave her for a few minutes so that she can calm down

B.   Ask her to put her complaints in writing

C.   Make her understand that it is not in your power to discuss the resident's care

D.   Listen to their complaints calmly and assure her of your readiness to discuss the same with the nurse

Answer is D

The best approach here will be to listen to such complaints and get them across to the nurse. Other options may not be adequate to calm the situation or raise any hope of resolution of such cases.

Question 17

When you urge a resident to take part in their care and related activities, you are improving their emotional and mental health needs by:

A. relieving the burden on you as a caregiver, considering the several tasks you have to complete

B. enhancing their sense of outlook, while making them more independent

C. holding them responsible for completing tasks

D. increasing their reliability

Answer is B

Residents who solely depend on others for the most little assistance gradually lose their independence, and subsequently their personality and outlook.

Thus, when you have them take part in their care and related activities, no matter how significant it may be, it is enough to improve their mood significantly.

Question 18

A resident that resents his family members has such feeling because:

A.   He thinks he has been abandoned by being left in a care facility

B.   He misses the annual birthday parties of the family

C.   He experiences spiritual unrest by his inability to attend church with his family

D.   He misses the usual family meals

Answer is A

Each option above is capable of contributing to resentment; the most common and usual of them is residents feeling abandoned when they consider the family's decision to transfer them to a care facility, thus putting their care in the hands of strangers.

Question 19

Empathy is an important caring characteristic that a nursing assistant must have to enable them to take care of the residents properly. 'Empathy' here is best defined as:

A. Being conscious of your comments and its effects on others

B. Being attentive enough to understand the cause of any negative reaction

C. Putting yourself in others' shoes without pitying them

D. All of these

Answer is D

Every option above clearly defines empathy, thus making it a top characteristic that a caregiver can portray.

Question 20

How would you approach a case of a sudden change in the mental condition of a resident?

A.   By spending more time with him or her as they may require more than the usual assistance

B.   By informing the charge nurse immediately of such changes

C.   By attempting to lighten up the mood of the resident by being humorous and funny

D.   By asking if the resident has also discovered any change in their personality

Answer is B

A change in the mental condition of a resident warrants an immediate report and action; a delay could cause something more serious while the quick report may prevent any further damage. Asking the resident if the change is evident to them may not always work, as they may be unaware of the change as well. While being humorous can help the situation, it should never be an alternative to reporting changes in mental condition.

CNA PRACTICE TEST 8

(35 Questions)

Question 1

One of the following are cases of neglect except?

A.   Leaving the clutter lying around the walkway

B.   Not providing the resident with the right amount of water as and when due

C.   Not moving an immovable resident enough so that they do not get bed sores

D.   Leaving the floor after having clocked in

Answer is D

Option D is not right, as a nurse assistant may have to leave the floor for different purposes during their shift. Failure in any of the situations described in the other options is a case of neglect.

Question 2

What best describes a situation where a charge nurse administered a prescribed medication to the wrong patient?

A. Malpractice
B. Assault
C. Battery
D. Neglect

Answer is A

Failure to execute medical duties as expected, and which eventually harms the patient is referred to as Nursing Malpractice. Other options are legal terms that are not adequate to describe this situation.

Question 3

A situation where a nursing assistant threatens to hit a resident that has refused to stop yelling is regarded as:

A. Assault
B. Battery
C. Slander
D. Libel

Answer is A

Assault is right here, as the situation is a reflection of a threat of harm. If the situation is an actual infliction of harm, it would be a battery. Libel and slander are only applicable in situations of verbal assaults against the character of someone.

Question 4

On welcoming the family of a resident you care for, one of the members offers you an envelope containing a "Thank You" complimentary card alongside some money, as a form of appreciation for your care towards their loved one. How would you deal with this situation?

A. Take the gift first and ask your colleagues about the best way to handle such situations later

B. Take the gift from them and increase the attention you give to this resident as a means of showing that you appreciate the gift

C. Appreciate the kind gesture of the family and use the money to get the resident a gift on his or her birthday

D. Appreciate the kind gesture of the family and the resident, but decline the gift pending the time you can check with the facility policies or your supervisor on the conditions of taking gifts in the facility

Answer is D

So far you are employed as a caregiver, it is against your professional ethics to accept monetary or other gifts from a resident or their family. In some facilities, such gifts may have to be donated to a fund that buys items for the use of every resident in the facility. However, note that policies on gifts differ across facilities. Problems may also arise when you take gifts from dementia patients.

Question 5

You just saw a contained fire in one of the rooms where residents reside. What would you do first as a nursing assistant?

A. Reach for the fire extinguisher

B. Get the residents in the room to safety

C. Immediately pull the fire alarm

D. Cry out for help immediately

Answer is B

The safety of residents remains the priority in cases of fire.

Question 6

A nursing assistant charged with battery must have done which of the following?

A. Threatening to slap a resident by raising his or her hand

B. Intentionally delaying the response to the call for help by a resident

C. Administering medications

D. Applying restraining devices on residents without directives from the physician

Answer is D

Putting residents on restraints without the approval of the physician is battery.

Question 7

A nursing assistant charged with negligence must have committed which of these offenses?

A. Pinching a resident's forehead while trimming their bangs

B. Failure to turn a patient after two hours as prescribed to prevent them from pressure sores

C. Failing to check on a patient intentionally at a stipulated time

D. Intentionally harming a resident by applying too much force

Answer is D

When you deliberately harm a resident, it is a physical abuse as well as battery. Other offenses in the list are all cases of negligence.

Question 8

Due to their anger towards you, a fellow nursing aide lied against you to the charge nurse that you stole from the bag of a resident. Such a situation can be described as:

A.   Accolades
B.   Defamation
C.   Malpractice
D.   Assault

Answer is B

Defamation refers to making false, usually offensive statements, about someone. Malpractice is an unlawful or unethical behavior that led to a failure to fulfill official duties expected of a position.

Question 9

A situation where a charge nurse informs the resident that the LPN is malfunctioning can be described legally as:

A. Slander
B. Insubordination
C. Discrimination
D. Gossip

Answer is A

Slander means uttering malicious statements capable of destroying the reputation of another person, while an unfair treatment of someone as a result of prejudice is termed discrimination. When a subordinate refuses to take orders, it is insubordination. In this situation, the charge nurse has gossiped, but gossip here is not a legal term.

Question 10

The statement - "being responsible for providing care according to the stipulations of an accepted standard," can be described legally as:

A. Slander
B. Liability
C. Legality
D. Aiding and abetting

Answer is B

Liability is the correct description of this situation. All other options have different legal meanings.

Question 11

A situation where a nursing assistant harasses a resident right in your presence, but you failed to report such, is referred to as:

A. Libel

B. Passive aggression
C. Aiding and abetting
D. Cease and desist

Answer is C

Choosing not to report a violation of a resident's right by a caregiver is considered aiding and abetting or contributing to an offense. Cease and desist refers to a demand to stop doing an allegedly illegal activity now and in the future.

Question 12

Without proper authorization, a nursing assistant decided on her own to restrict the actions or movement of a resident. How would you describe such a situation?

A. Slander
B. Liability

C. Aiding and abetting

D. False imprisonment

Answer is D

Using restraints without the approval of a physician is not the only action that is considered to be false imprisonment and violation of the rights of a resident, threatening to restrain patients against their approval and that of the physician can lead to charges of false imprisonment.

Question 13

The act of forcing a patient to do something against their will can be classified as:

A. Consequences

B. Conspiracy

C. Coercion

D. Collusion

Answer is C

Any secret plot or plan by two or more individuals is referred to as a conspiracy. The aftermath of a particular behavior, usually unacceptable, are termed consequences. When people engage in secret cooperation to do something illegal, it is called collusion.

Question 14

Involuntary seclusion is represented by which of the following?

A.   Giving a resident some privacy when they want to speak with their family

B.   Leaving a patient on their own without adequate communication devices, like the call bell

C.   Leaving the door of a patient closed once they request for a private time

D. Carrying a patient from their bed to the wheelchair and driving them away when they ask for some private time

Answer is B

When a patient is deprived of his means of communication while alone, it is a case of involuntary seclusion because the patient never wanted such a situation. All other cases are what the patient requested for.

Question 15

What would you do if a resident starts complaining of thirst and hunger on his return from a day trip with his family members?

A. Tell the resident the family who was in charge assured you they had strictly followed mealtime schedules

B. Tell the resident when the next snack and beverage time is scheduled and get him or her a glass of water

C. Talk to the family about the importance of the resident getting proper snacks when on an outing

D. Inform the nurse of such development

Answer is D

Any suspected abuse, by fellow residents, family members, or even friends, must be immediately reported to the nursing charge.

Question 16

An example of a situation that violates the resident's right is:

A. A patient is being treated by a physician that they have asked to be dismissed

B. Putting a resident on restraint after they tried to punch a nurse giving him care

C. Changing the clothes of a resident by a nursing assistant, from their "lucky shirt" to the hospital gown, because the former is soiled and stinking

D. Transferring a patient from a standard facility to one with reduced functionality because of the inability of the patient to pay the bills

Answer is A

According to the Bill of Rights of patients, patients are allowed to work with their preferred physician. Concerning restraints, a doctor's order overrules the wish of the patient to wear them or not.

Question 17

Which of these would be an example of invasion of a patient's privacy?

A. Exposing the resident's body unnecessarily when performing his or her care

B. Not shutting the resident's door when exiting the room

C. Discussing the resident's dislikes with a co-worker while reporting

D. Refusal to knock on a patient's door before entering

Answer is A

Not keeping the affairs of residents confidential or exposing their body unnecessarily during care is considered an invasion of privacy. It is always advisable to knock before entering a resident's room, although failing to do so is not an invasion of privacy. Unless asked to do so by the resident, it is not necessary to shut the door when exiting the room. Lastly, sharing confidential information during a report is necessary for patient care, but should be done in an area in which nonessential medical staff or other residents cannot overhear this information.

Question 18

A liability is defined as:

A. The unavailability of care of acceptable standards

B. Being responsible for caring according to standards

C. Having poor knowledge of how to execute duties correctly and professionally

D. Taking part in illegal acts

Answer is B

Being responsible for caring according to acceptable standards is called competency. When a nursing assistant performs duties outside his or her job description appropriately, or perform appropriate duties wrongly and thus harming a resident, it may lead to charges of liability.

Question 19

Which of these is not an example of abuse?

A. Kicking a resident

B. Threatening to hit a resident

C. Hitting a resident

D. Doing things that startle a resident

Answer is D

When you threaten a resident or execute an actual physical or mental harm on a resident, it is an abuse. Although startling residents may cause a considerable level of anxiety, such do not last for long and is not considered as an act or threat of abuse.

Question 20

All of these are liable acts, except?

A.   abuse

B.   invading people's privacy

C.   theft

D.   voluntary seclusion

Answer is D

All of the options are liable acts (including involuntary seclusion), except involuntary seclusion. When you prevent a resident from associating with others as a means of punishing them, it is an involuntary seclusion, but when they request for it themselves, it is a voluntary seclusion.

Question 21

An order reads thus: Using a "passive range of motion" exercises only, increase the muscle strength and joint mobility of the resident in question. As a nursing assistant who is to carry out the order, how would you proceed?

A.   Have the resident move his or her arm in a circular direction at short time intervals

B.   Have the resident lift objects that are not heavy at short intervals

C.   Hold the arm of the resident carefully, while smoothly moving it circularly

D.   Put the arm of the patient through resistance exercises

Answer is C

The phrase "passive range of motion," as used concerning the exercises above, explains the types of exercises performed on an individual who cannot move limbs voluntarily. The other options assume that the resident in question can voluntarily maneuver on their own.

Question 22

When inadequate body mechanics are used, injuries are inevitable. Which of these muscles is most susceptible to such injuries?

A. Muscles of the arm
B. Muscles of the back
C. Muscles of the leg
D. Muscles of the neck

Answer is B

The muscles of the lower back are the most prone to injuries arising from improper body mechanics. All other options highlighted are additional areas of injury.

Question 23

If you want to encourage the independence of a resident, which of the following would you do as a resident?

A. Cleaning the resident up only a when they have been soiled, with the hope that they will be encouraged to go to the bathroom on their own

B. Having the resident start the morning care routine and assisting only when it is needed

C. Having the resident's roommates assist one another in the course of their morning care routine

D. Leaving the room after providing the resident with the required items for the morning care routine, so that he or she may be motivated to start without assistance

Answer is B

As a nursing assistant, you must leave some duties to the residents to handle on their own. However, you should be ready to assist once they need one, especially concerning some tough tasks. One could view the other options as a form of neglect.

Question 24

Which of the following is not a function of an assisting device?

A. Moving around
B. Restraining
C. Dressing
D. Eating

Answer is B

Assisting devices such as canes, reaching rods, braces, and splints are products that make tasks and activities easier to perform. Restraining does the opposite and impedes movement.

Question 25

If you are to give care to a resident that has a rehabilitation plan of care, what would be your role as the nursing assistant?

A. Reduce the time given to residents to complete tasks with the view of speeding up their recovery

B. Provide more than the usual assistance to residents in completing their tasks

C. Helping with retaining

D. Administering pain medications

Answer is C

Rehabilitation plans are to help residents regain the ability to do tasks they were able to do before being disabled. This may involve retraining old skills or introducing new ways of doing things to return functioning to normal as much as possible.

Administering pain medications, decreasing what a resident does, or pressuring

Question 26

The definition: "Nursing interventions that promote the resident's ability to adapt and adjust to living as independently and safely as possible," best describes:

A. Restorative Nursing
B. Occupational Nursing
C. Therapeutic Nursing
D. Proactive Nursing

Answer is A

Restorative Nursing is a defined area of nursing that goes beyond rehabilitation. Some normal function may never be recoverable, and the patient may need behavioral or cognitive activities that help him or her learn how to deal with an issue that is unrecoverable. The other choices are not defined areas of nursing like Restorative Nursing, but they may be involved in the process of restoration.

Question 27

As a nursing assistant, how would you assist a resident that you are helping with ambulation who experiences pain while using splints?

A.   Making them know that the pains are a result of overdoing the therapy, and thus they should reduce their time on the floor

B.   Making them understand that the pain is normal and will leave once they adjust to the splint

C.   Administer topical pain medication on the affected areas

D.   Inform the charge nurse immediately

Answer is D

A situation like a painful splint use should be tabled before the charge nurse as soon as possible, as this might signify the presence of more serious issues that require prompt attention. A nursing assistant must not consider all other options; they do more harm and no good.

Question 28

A resident who also works with a physical therapist has been told to engage in some "range of motion" activities. As the nursing assistant giving care to him, what do you understand by such a directive?

A. Give the resident hygiene care

B. Give the resident spiritual and cultural care

C. Give the patient restorative care

D. Give the patient emotional and mental care

Answer is C

The range of motion activities are used as a therapy to restore or maintain mobility and flexibility and are an important component of restorative care. The other answers are incorrect.

Question 29

Which of the following complications arising from immobility can be reduced or prevented using restorative care?

A. Labored breathing
B. Hypotension
C. Dry skin
D. Clotting of the blood

Answer is D

Clotting of the blood is a severe complication arising from immobility, and it can be prevented via restorative nursing.

Question 30

"To turn upward" defines which of these terms?

A. Lateral
B. Eversion
C. Supination
D. Extension

Answer is C

By supination, we mean turning upward. Lateral, here, is wrong as it means "to the side," while extension refers to straightening, and eversion, turning outward.

Question 31

The best instance of restorative care skills is:

A. Using a denture soaking dish

B. Applying heating pads for stiff necks

C. Applying adult briefs or pads for conditions of incontinence

D. Using therapeutic, assistive, and adaptive equipment as required

Answer is D

The best instance is the use of therapeutic, assistive, and adaptive equipment as required. Although the other options pass for routine cares, they do not come out as the best answer for defining restorative care.

Question 32

In restorative care, it is vital to understand common disease processes and conditions because?

A. They may slow down the progress of the care

B.   They influence the functions of the body system concerning the aptitude for success with restorative care on the resident

C.   Such knowledge influences the type of care management that will be considered as appropriate

D.   All of these reasons are right

Answer is D

All the reasons highlighted above are correct concerning having proper knowledge of disease processes and conditions.

Question 33

Muscle wasting is medically termed as

A.   Atrophy

B.   Hypoxia

C.   Shrivel

D.   Anorexia

Answer is A

The correct medical term to define muscles that waste away is "atrophy." Unusual loss of appetite is termed anorexia, while deficiency of oxygen that gets to the tissues is termed hypoxia.

Question 34

PROM means:

A. Positive Reversing Motion

B. Passive Range of Motion

C. Positioning References on Machines

D. Positive Range of Motivation

Answer is B

The term "passive range of motion" is used to explain "assisted" motions, and it functions in the prevention of atrophy, enhancing circulation, and creating mobility.

Question 35

How can you differentiate abduction from adduction?

A. Movement towards and from the body; abduction moves the extremity towards, while adduction moves it away

B. Adduction moves only an extremity, while abduction moves the entire body

C. Adduction can be done with a single person, while two or more persons are required for abduction

D. Adduction means moving the extremity towards the body, while abduction means moving it far away from the body

Answer is D

Adduction means moving an extremity towards the body, while abduction is the direct opposite, i.e., moving an extremity away from the body.

CONCLUSION

Thank you for purchasing this book!

Like most professional examinations, the CNA Examinations also require adequate preparation, in addition to excellent professional experience.

This book has been structured to give prospective participants in the CNA Examinations a clear insight into what to expect in the written portion of the exams.

Each question in this book has been carefully selected, and adequately answered to ensure that the reader not only understands each question but also why the answer is preferred to other options.

Thus, as a candidate, if you have taken time peruse the questions, then you have very high chances of coming out successful in your CNA Examinations.

Thank you once again and Good luck!

www.ingramcontent.com/pod-product-compliance
Lightning Source LLC
Chambersburg PA
CBHW031826170526
45157CB00001B/196